STARTING YOGA

A Practical Foundation Guide
for Men and Women

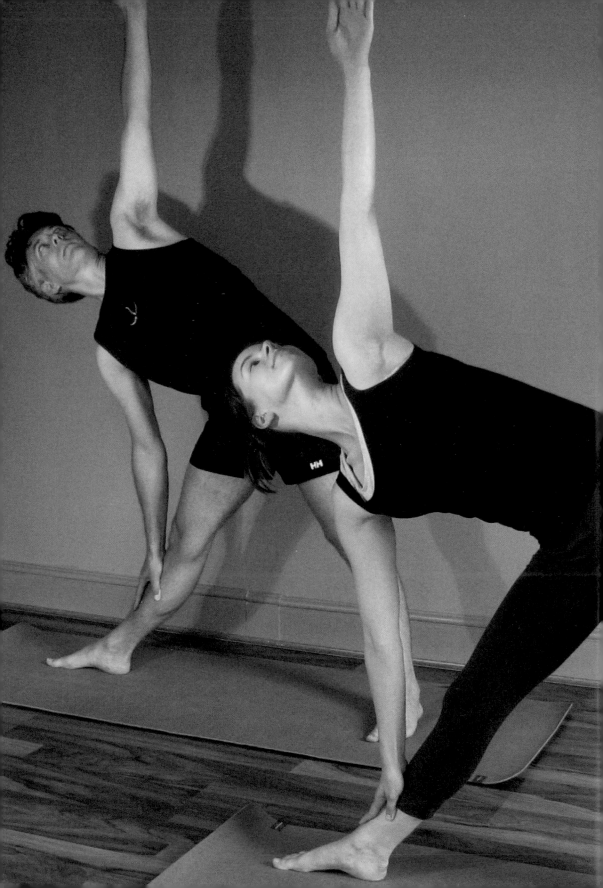

STARTING YOGA

A Practical Foundation Guide
for Men and Women

Alan Bradbury

THE CROWOOD PRESS

First published in 2011 by
The Crowood Press Ltd
Ramsbury, Marlborough
Wiltshire SN8 2HR

www.crowood.com

British Library Cataloguing-in-Publication Data
A catalogue record for this book is available from the British Library.

ISBN 978 1 84797 241 5

Disclaimer
Whilst every effort has been made to ensure that the content of this book is
as technically accurate as possible, neither the author nor the publishers can
accept responsibility for any injury or loss sustained as a result of the use
of the material contained in this publication. It is the responsibility of the
individual to ensure that they are fit to participate and they should seek
medical advice from a qualified professional before undertaking any Yoga
training or exercises of any kind.

Designed and typeset by Focus Publishing,
11a St Botolph's Road, Sevenoaks, Kent TN13 3AJ

Printed and bound in Singapore by Craft Print International Ltd.

Contents

Foreword *by Dr Alberto Albeniz*

I met Alan five years ago, having tested two other different yoga classes. I finally decided to stay with him. What was it that made me stay? On reflection, this decision was facilitated by several factors.

Firstly, I felt attracted by his approach, which combined small talks and debates about principles of yoga philosophy with a substantial demonstration and deepening through a gradually planned series of yoga postures. There it was, a man in his sixties modelling his preach. Secondly, a mixture of sense of humour and laissez-fair encouragement that was all the time respectful of the students' needs and limitations. Thirdly, despite yoga being a traditional male ancient activity, nowadays it seemed to be dominated by women. This sometimes could be slightly overpowering for shy men like me. To my glad surprise, his classes had that comfortable touch that related to men and women students of all ages.

Finally, I found that after a hectic and often stressful and professional day at work as a consultant psychiatrist and psychotherapist in the NHS, I experienced while walking back home after his class some enjoyable aliveness in my body coupled with a resting awareness.

Alan is a family man originally from Manchester. His background includes lecturing in orthodontics at Leeds University Dental Institute. Perhaps this explains his didactic skills and his fidelity to scientific principles. On the other hand, his humanistic approach stands out. Alan has relentlessly studied and practised yoga since 1973 and has developed an eclectic style. He has trained as a yoga teacher with The British Wheel of Yoga and has studied Iyengar Yoga with Kristal Clark in Leeds and at The Iyengar Institute of South London.

Foundation books usually fall into the trap of either simplifying messages too naively or putting people off unnecessarily through complex concepts or practice. His book is an achievement in the necessary balance of fitting the beginners' needs for simplicity, clarity and guidance with the accessibility and loyalty to the traditional philosophical elements. Alan capitalizes on his innate communication skills through a mixture of narrative and pictures that are coherent and easy to follow and convey the fundamental principles in which Hatha Yoga is based. He is clearly not aiming or claiming to change people's lives. But this book beautifully reproduces what in my personal experience I have consistently witnessed in his class: a subtle influence that improves quality of life. His book reflects his gentle and elegant style with his natural and infectious liking of people.

I welcome you to enjoy this book and allow yourself to test its teachings with real life practice.

Dr Alberto Albeniz
LMS, MRCPsych, Memb IGA
Stratford-upon-Avon

Acknowledgements

This book could not have been possible without the expertise, generosity, kindness and support of friends, relatives and colleagues who when asked to take part in this project readily gave their talents with energy and commitment.

I am indebted to my brother, Dr Vic Bradbury, who so adeptly and patiently produced the photographs which brought the text to life. I should also like to thank Katherine Sanders for the lovely additional photographs taken outdoors. I express my gratitude to my two dedicated models Stephanie Bradbury and Paul Walton who willingly and enthusiastically gave their time and skill during the long photo shoot.

I could not have managed without the technical support of Ben White. Not only is he a kind and generous being, he is a clever computer scientist. His contribution has been invaluable.

My heartfelt thanks are offered to Allan Oakman, my first yoga teacher, the man who kindled my interest in yoga in the 1970s and whose spirit and enthusiasm remain with me to date. Thanks also to Kristal Clark my Iyengar teacher in Leeds. She kept my fire alight and guided me along the path with such skill and dedication. To Yoga Masters BKS Iyengar and Godfrey Devereux I am eternally thankful. They have continually aroused my passion for yoga through their inspiring books so full of wisdom and expertise. And not least, I am indebted to the support of my students who have been a continual source of inspiration, making my journey at all times enjoyable and worthwhile.

I was indeed fortunate to make contact with The Crowood Press, whose staff have been a tower of help and support. I thank them sincerely for all their expertise in making the publication of my book a reality.

Finally, I offer my deepest appreciation and love to my wife Josephine. She is the one who has kept my spirit alive during the writing of this book. Her encouragement, practical advice, constant faith, wisdom, emotional support and not least sense of humour have been a never-failing source of strength and to her I dedicate this book.

Introduction

This book is based on the teachings of my Foundation Course in yoga, which is aimed at complete beginners and also those who may have dabbled with yoga in the past and wish to rekindle their interest. My aim is to make it simple and accessible whilst at the same time giving full service to the fundamental principles.

The intention is to get you started on the path of yoga and to spark your interest in what is a vast subject with a long and fascinating history and which has become very popular worldwide. I hope it will give you, as it did me, the opportunity to experience some of the wonderful benefits that yoga can provide. I became hooked on yoga in the 1970s when I joined a local authority evening class and had the good fortune to meet a wonderful yoga teacher, Allan Oakman, whose enthusiasm and spirit remain with me to the present day. Since then I have practised yoga almost every day and over the years have had the opportunities to meet and work with some excellent yoga teachers; my students have also been a continual source of joy. It is something I can wholeheartedly recommend.

Yoga is the oldest form of mind and body fitness. Originating in India thousands of years ago, it is now accepted worldwide as a recognized system of mental and physical training. The word yoga means 'union' and as such can be interpreted as the joining together of mind, body and spirit. Yoga is essentially about balance. The world is rapidly changing and life can be challenging in our technological age. To remain steady and focused in the midst of the whirlpool of life is becoming increasingly difficult and yoga offers a way of coping. Being fit and healthy in body and mind gives the opportunity for greater contentment so that we can enjoy a full life in all its complexity.

Whilst it is easy to become complacent, settling for what we have and refusing to budge from our habits and conditioned ways, it can be exciting to take on a new challenge. What is best for most of us is finding the right balance in life. And in a way this sums up the process of yoga: it is about finding balance, satisfying our fundamental need to feel safe and secure, yet at the same time being prepared to venture beyond our comfort zones and feel free. There are various reasons why we are drawn to yoga. It may be that we simply want to get fit or fitter. We may want to reduce our stress level, sleep better, or tackle a weight problem. We may be encouraged to take up yoga by a friend or partner. Whatever our motive we all want to feel good about ourselves. Yoga is for everyone, regardless of age or level of fitness, offering a way of finding our potential and ultimately of knowing who we are. This route to self-realization is not about competition, or success or failure, but about wanting to experience life to the full with all its ups and downs, highs and lows.

How to Use This Book

It is best that you become familiar with the principles of yoga practice before you start and it may be wise to read the book first to enable you to get a feel for the subject. When you are ready, you may prefer to work quietly on your own or with a friend or partner. You might wish to use the book in combination with attending a yoga class. I hope you will find the course straightforward and it is by no means intended to take you to an advanced level. Yet, as in most things that are worthwhile and have lasting benefits, a strong foundation of firm understanding is vital for a satisfying and fruitful progression.

The yoga postures I have chosen represent some of the classical postures you will find in most yoga classes. They are by no means exhaustive (there are hundreds of different postures). Allow yourself to be selective. If any of the postures do not feel right or are too strenuous, then feel free to leave them out of your routine – you can always return to them later. Work steadily, allowing sufficient time to become familiar with one posture before moving on to the next. Bear in mind that your yoga practice is for you alone and although some discipline is required, you are not trying to conform to a standard. Flexibility, muscular strength, body type and so on are determined to a large extent by our genes and we each have our own needs and limitations. So be prepared to enjoy the process and to experience the benefits without comparison to others.

1 Getting Started

You will need your own space, ideally a warm, airy room. The basic equipment is a yoga mat, two yoga blocks and a yoga belt. These can be purchased quite cheaply from many sports retailers or via the Internet from one of the yoga suppliers. A blanket will also be useful. Then all that is required is a little discipline and a regular time to practise. Most of us have hectic lives, but avoid the common misconception of being too busy to find time to practise regularly. By becoming fitter, healthier and more focused, your efficiency level improves and you will have more energy. Consequently, your coping skills will receive a boost, enhancing your enjoyment and productivity whether it is in your work, your leisure or your family life.

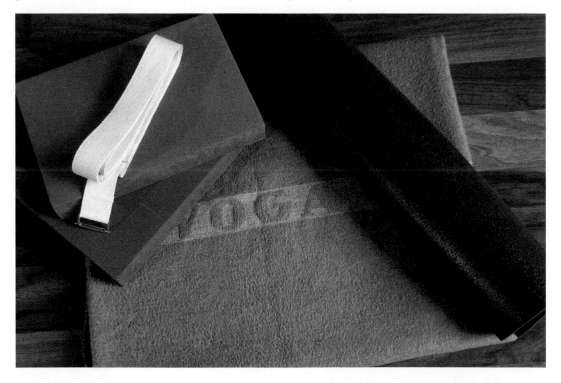

Basic equipment.

Medical conditions and precautions

You should always consult your doctor before embarking on a course of a physical nature. This is essential if you have a pre-existing medical condition. The British Wheel of Yoga[1] recognizes certain medical conditions which require the supervision of a qualified yoga teacher. These include: heart conditions; uncontrolled blood pressure problems; glaucoma/eye disorders; hernias and ulcers; pregnancy; spine conditions; arthritis; respiratory disorders and mental conditions. Once you get your doctor's approval you will need to seek out a qualified yoga teacher as some of the postures in the book may not be suitable for you. A yoga teacher can modify the postures making them safe to practise at home.

Yoga is not suitable for anyone who has had a recent abdominal operation.

This book is not intended for women who are pregnant. If you are pregnant or have recently given birth, you should consult a yoga teacher who specializes in Yoga for Pregnancy.

Preparation for your practice

Here are a few helpful hints in preparing for your practice:
- It is best not to eat a big meal for a couple of hours before your practice. A small snack will not be harmful.
- Women should avoid strenuous work and certain postures during menstruation.
- Where possible, try to practice in the same place and at the same time of day, at a time when you will not be disturbed.
- It is better to do a short practice regularly than a longer practice inconsistently.

The yoga session has structure. It is usual to start with a period of calm, either sitting quietly or lying on your back. The purpose of this is to settle your mind and body to allow you to release from the daily pressures and to move into your practice in a steady and focused way. This is followed by stretching exercises to warm and loosen up your body in preparation for the yoga postures which are the main part. The session is concluded with a short period of calm so that you leave your practice feeling refreshed and relaxed.

Yoga postures

The yogic word for posture is 'asana', meaning 'seat' or 'position'. In yoga we assume specific positions with the intention of becoming stronger and more flexible. Yet this is purely physical training unless we look further: at a deeper level we are stimulating the flow of energy in the body to increase our vitality. We are also refreshing our internal organs as well as invigorating our bodily systems. And what distinguishes yoga from some of the more conventional methods of physical training is the expression of mind/body integration. In yoga we continually remind ourselves to bring full attention and awareness to the sensations in our body and to our breath and to whatever we are experiencing in the moment. This involves being focused and steady throughout our practice so that we function holistically. Frank Jude Boccio[2] succinctly refers to cultivating the potential of 'mindfulness' through our asana practice. He clarifies mindfulness as:

> ...the practice of continuously remembering to stay present, not losing ourselves in forgetfulness of where we are, what we are doing, and whom we are with. Mindfulness is always arising in relationship – to ourselves, including our breath, body movements and feelings and to our surroundings and all we experience physically, mentally and emotionally.

The enhanced awareness that develops through yoga helps us to recognize when we are holding tension in our body. Tension may be caused by emotional problems past or present, or through years of careless habits resulting in faulty posture. Unless we recognize and correct these habits, they will remain as obstacles to our becoming fitter and healthier and may manifest as problems as we get older such as bad backs and painful joints. And being fit and healthy brings confidence and a sense of freedom.

The changes you will experience through your yoga practice are subtle and you need to explore the postures carefully without trying to push ahead too quickly.

The skeletal system

It will be helpful at this stage to gain some insight into the body's skeletal system. Knowledge of the anatomy of the skeleton will help you to perceive the correct alignment of your body. A well-aligned skeleton is essential to good posture.

The spine as the central and vertical axis of the body is the key structure. A healthy spine suggests a healthy body. The spine runs vertically, connecting with the base of the skull at the top and with the pelvis below. See how the head is balanced centrally with the chin in line with the notch at the top of the breastbone (sternum). The lower part of the spine, the sacrum, is fused with the pelvis and ends in the tail bone (coccyx). Observe the pelvis: this is the largest and heaviest bone in the body. We refer to the circular projections at the base of the pelvis as the 'sitting bones'. The thigh bones (femurs) connect with the pelvis on each side at the pelvic joints. Follow the lines of the legs from the pelvic joints to the knee joints, from the knee joints into the ankle joints and into the feet and toes.

Observe the rib cage, which surrounds the chest and encloses and protects the heart and lungs. The twelve pairs of ribs are attached at the back to the spinal vertebrae and surround the chest cavity to connect at the front with the sternum (with the exception of the two lowest ribs, known as 'floating ribs'). The collar bones (clavicles) connect on each side with the top of the sternum and run horizontally to join the upper arms forming part of the shoulder girdle. The shoulder blades (scapulae) which are situated behind the rib cage complete the shoulder girdle. Follow the lines of the arms from shoulder joints to the elbow joints, from elbows into the wrist joints and into the hands and fingers.

The area between the bottom of the rib cage and the pubic bone at the base of the pelvis is the abdomen.

Now look at the spine in side view. The spine comprises thirty-three vertebrae which, with the exception of the lower nine vertebrae which are fused, are each separated by a joint and a spinal disc. From the side aspect we can see the natural curvatures of the spine. In the neck region there is a mild inwards curve (cervical spine). The spine then curves gently outwards in the upper back (thoracic spine). The curve is again inwards in the lower back (lumbar spine), then outwards at the sacrum which fuses with the pelvis. The spine terminates at the tail bone (coccyx) in a final inwards curve.

Spend a little time studying the skeleton, observing the structures, joints, alignment and symmetry.

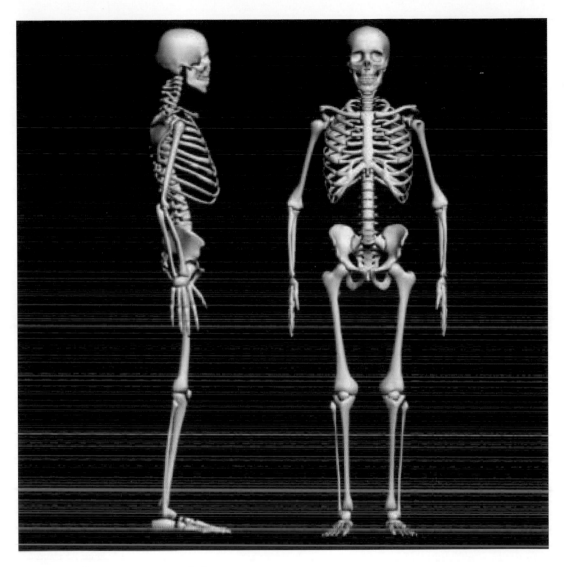

Anatomically correct human skeleton.

2   Starting Your Practice

Many of the yoga postures take their names from nature, representing animals, vegetation, mythological beings and universal phenomena. Traditionally, the names of the postures are written and spoken in Sanskrit, the ancient and sacred language of India. I shall use the more familiar English descriptions.

The Corpse Pose

The Corpse Pose involves simply lying down on your back 'as still as a corpse'. This posture can be useful at the start of your practice to enable you to settle down and de-stress. It is also beneficial for winding down at the end of your practice.

1. Sit on your mat. With bent knees, take the palms of your hands behind you (fingers pointing forwards) and lean back taking your weight onto your palms.
2. Ease gently down onto your elbows and fore-arms and look along the line of your body to make sure you are not lying at an angle.

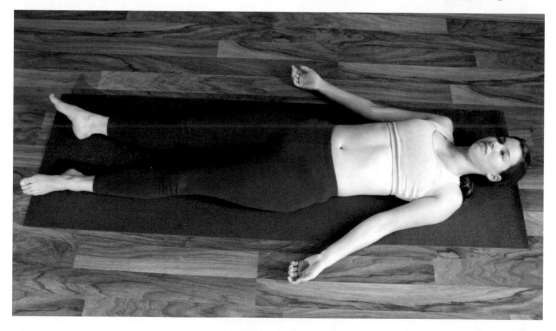

The Corpse Pose.

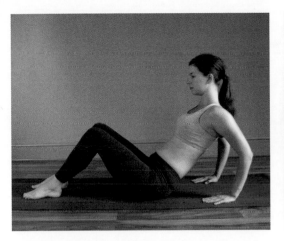

1.

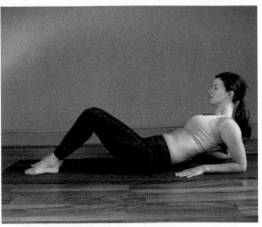

2.

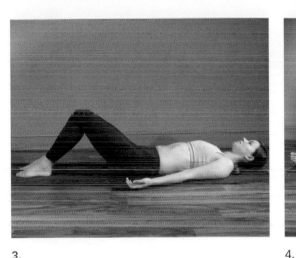

3.

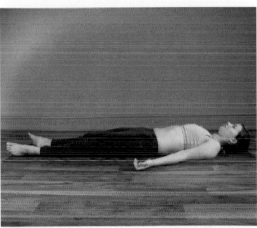

4.

3. Gently release onto your back. Position your head centrally so that your chin is level with the notch at the top of your breastbone. Keep your chin tucked in slightly so that your throat is relaxed and the back of your neck assumes its length and natural inward curve. Relax your shoulders, moving them down away from your ears and roll them gently back towards the mat so that your chest is full and broad. Extend your arms by your sides taking them at an angle of approxi-mately ten degrees away from your trunk with palms facing upwards. Focus on your spine in the midline of your back. Lift your pelvis slightly and push it towards your heels. This will help lengthen your lower back and adjust the lumbar curve.

4. Allow your pelvis and back to settle on the mat before straightening your legs. Keep your heels close and allow the balls of your feet to roll gently out to the sides. You are now in the full Corpse Pose.

Modification: If the chin tends to stick up (see Fig. 5), there will be tension in the throat muscles and pressure on the vertebrae in the neck. In which case, it will be necessary to rest the back of your head on a block to achieve the right balance (see Fig. 6).

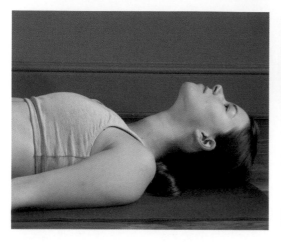

5.

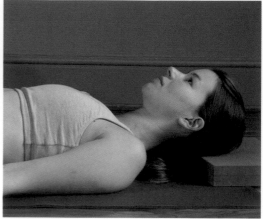

6.

Relaxing in Corpse Pose

Envisage the symmetry of your posture. With the spine as the central axis, the right and left sides of your body should mirror image each other. Be your own witness and observe how you are feeling both mentally and physically. Fully embrace these feelings. Feel the contact of your back and the weight of your body on the mat. Embrace the feelings of being stable and supported on the firm ground. Take a few moments to feel that you are 'grounded'. In contrast, allow the feelings of lightness and ease to infiltrate the surface of your body. Let the muscles of your face soften and relax, particularly your eyes, tongue root and lower jaw. If you are clenching your teeth, allow them to slightly separate. Feel as if you are opening your heart and that your chest is becoming light and expansive. Relax your abdomen. Focus on your pelvis and release any tension you may be holding in the muscles of your pelvic floor. Allow the palms of your hands to soften and notice how your fingers lightly curl.

Focusing on the breath

Our breath is with us constantly although most of the time we do not think about our breathing. In yoga we deliberately bring our attention to our breath and this provides us with a vehicle for focus, which helps to steady and settle the mind.

1. Remain in the Corpse Pose. Bring your attention to your breath.
2. Focus on the sensation of air entering and leaving your nostrils as you breathe in and out. Notice the temperature of the air flowing along your nasal passages – it will be slightly warmer as you breathe out.
3. Do not attempt to analyze your breathing or change the rhythm – just say focused on the feel of the air as it flows in and out of your nasal passages. If you mind should wander, notice what distracted you and bring your attention back to your breath. It does not matter how often this occurs – just keep returning your attention to the feel of your breath.

The above is a simple yet effective technique for bringing steadiness to the mind. With regular practice, you will find that you become less vulnerable to the distractions of your surroundings. The enhanced level of conscious awareness that you develop by focusing on the breath intensifies the yoga process. It is when you feel balanced and steady that you get the full benefit. You will also gain an understanding of the concept of 'being in the moment' and come to realize the importance of the 'now'. So much of our time can be spent in thoughts of past events or thinking about the future, that it is easy to neglect what is going on in the present. The regular practice of bringing conscious awareness to the sensations in your body and to your breath will encourage the steadiness

and ease in body and mind which will allow you to experience what is happening right now. Your yoga training will come to influence your day-to-day experiences, giving you better control of your circumstances and more confidence and contentment.

The art of relaxation

To be relaxed, you need to learn how to let go of tension and resistance. It is about not 'holding on' to past events that may have affected you physically or emotionally, and not worrying unnecessarily about what might happen in the future. If we learn to embrace the present moment by tuning in to whatever we are experiencing – physically, mentally, emotionally – we will eventually find that we are able to 'let go'.

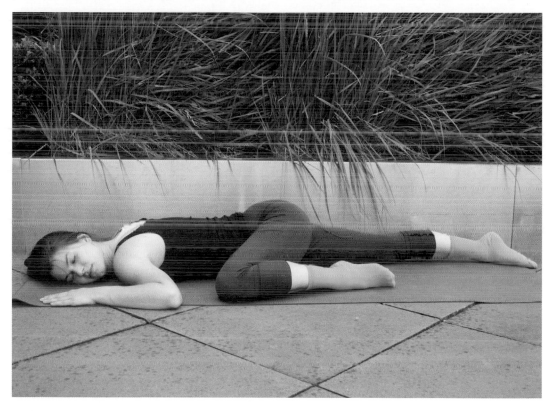

The joy of relaxation.

Stretching

The term 'supine' refers to lying on your back. The following exercises are described as supine stretches. They are effectively warm-up exercises as a preliminary to the yoga postures. The movements are coordinated with the breath and should be smooth and rhythmical. As a general rule, movements associated with opening and expanding the front of the body coincide with an in-breath and those which 'close' the front of the body with an out-breath. The ability to synchronize your breath and movements will improve with practice. Unless you have a nasal obstruction, always inhale and exhale through your nose. Inhaling brings energy and vitality to the body, whilst exhaling coincides with release and letting go.

Supine Arm Wave

1. Commence in Corpse Pose. Inhaling, raise your arms, taking them up and over behind your head. The start of your movement should coincide with the start of your in-breath; aim to have your arms stretched fully behind by the end of inhalation.

2. Exhale as you lower your arms to your sides. (Continue 'waving' your arms on the breath for several repetitions. You will soon pick up on the synchronization of your breath and movement. Pay attention to the sensations in your arms, shoulders and chest as you continue the arm wave.)

3. After several repetitions prepare to hold the stretch for several breaths. Spreading your palms, push gently into your finger-tips and push your toes away. Breathe freely and focus on the sensations as you extend your body. As you stretch, your abdominal wall will become longer and flatter, your chest full and broad. Notice the charges of energy along your arms and legs as you push into your fingers and toes. Now bring your toes towards you and push into your heels.

4. Clasp your fingers and placing the tips of your thumbs together, turn your palms to face the wall behind you and push into your palms whilst pushing your toes away once more. Change the clasp (see below) and continue the stretch. Exhaling, release your arms to your sides returning to Corpse Pose.

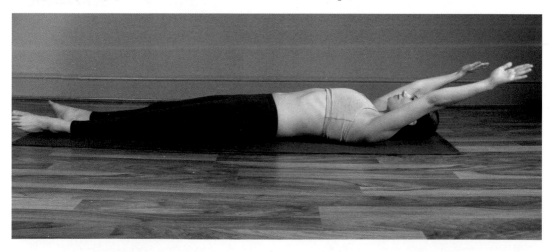

The Supine Arm Wave. 1.

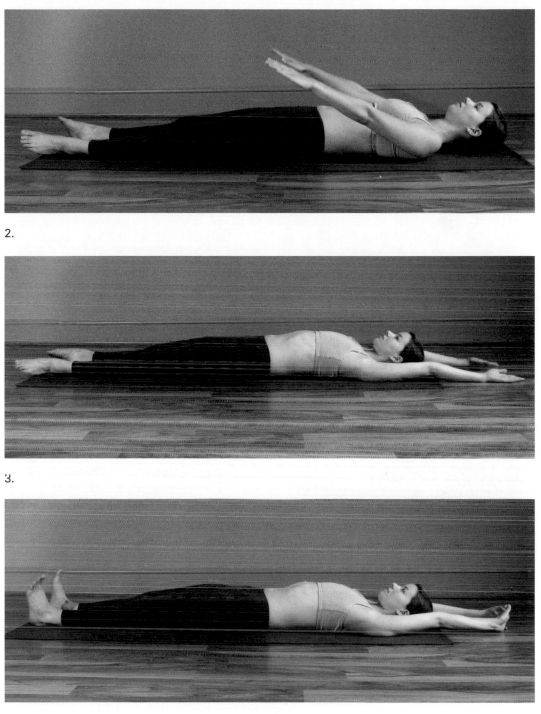

2.

3.

4.

Changing the clasp

Clasping your fingers and pushing your palms away from you stretches the muscles of your arms and brings flexibility to the wrists. By changing the position of your fingers part-way through the stretch, you harmonize the forces in your wrists and arms, thus maintaining a balanced stretch.

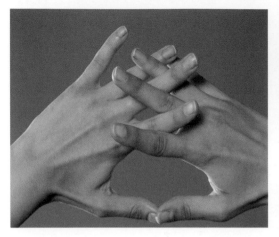 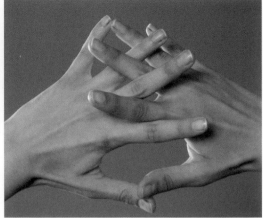

Changing the clasp. 1, 2.

Supine Leg Wave involving raising and lowering the legs alternately on the breath

1. Commence in Corpse Pose. Exhaling, raise your right leg at a comfortable angle to your pelvis. Keep your leg straight and bring your toes towards you gently pushing the sole of your foot away. Engage your leg muscles.

2. Lower the leg as you inhale.
   Repeat with the left leg then continue for several repetitions, maintaining a smooth rhythm and synchronizing your movement with your breath. Observe the physical sensations, paying particular attention to the charge of energy in the leg muscles. Take care to avoid strain.

Supine Leg Wave.

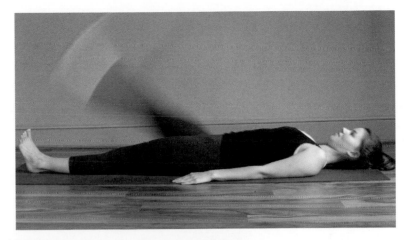

1.

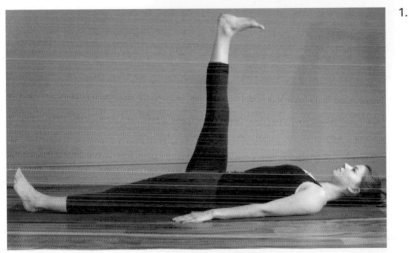

2.

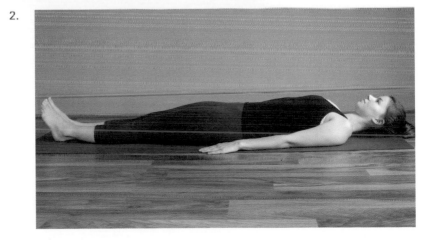

The Bridge Pose

This stretches the torso and awakens the spine.

1. Commence in Corpse Pose. Bend your knees and bring your heels in close to your pelvis. Your feet should be parallel and at hip width, with your knees resting above your heels and ankles.

2. Taking your weight into your heels, lift your pelvis off the mat. Push your pelvis upwards allowing your spine to arch gently into your back. Maintain the length in your tail bone and come up to rest on your shoulders and upper back, with your chin tucked in towards your sternum. Keep the weight in your heels and your face relaxed with your chest full, broad

The Bridge Pose.

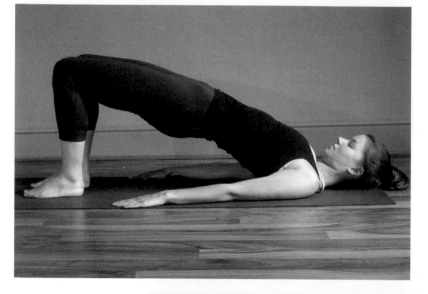

 1.

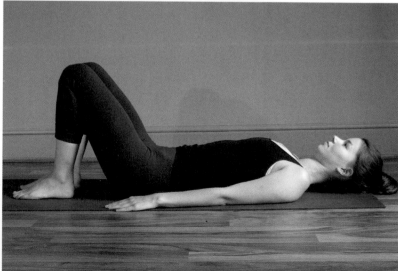

and active, your abdomen long and flat.

3. To release, curve your spine supporting it on the mat, vertebra by vertebra, all the way down from the upper back to the pelvis. Finally release your pelvis onto the mat.

Once you have mastered the technique, do three or four repetitions, moving up and down on the breath. Inhale as you move into the Bridge Pose and exhale as you release.

Caution: do not allow your abdomen to 'bloat', as this will cause exaggeration of your lumbar curve. Keeping your abdomen long, firm and flat gives support to your lower back.

2.

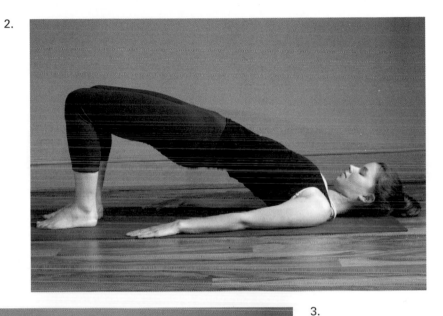

3.

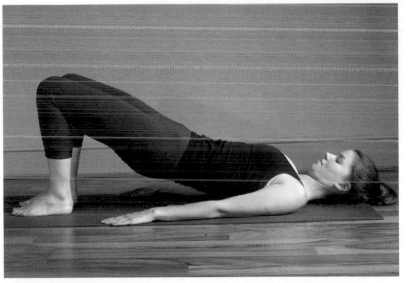

The Double Knee Wave

This helps to massage the lower back and tones the abdomen.

1. Commence in Corpse Pose. Bend both knees and lifting your feet, take hold of your knees in your hands, your elbows tucked in to your sides. Exhaling, squeeze your knees in towards your chest, keeping the back of your pelvis flat on the mat.

2. Inhale as you push your knees away from your face, allowing your elbows to extend.

Continue for several repetitions, maintaining a smooth rhythm on the breath. Each time you squeeze your knees in you will feel your lower back pressing into the mat and this will have a soothing effect.

The Double Knee Wave.

1.

2.

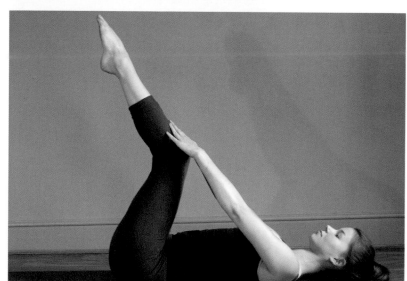

Releasing from the supine postures including Corpse Pose

1. Squeeze your knees towards your chest; gently lifting your head, rock back and forth on your spine.
2. If your back is strong enough, 'rock yourself up' to sitting position.
3. Alternatively, squeeze your knees in and roll over onto your side before bringing yourself up on hands and knees.

Caution: always be mindful of avoiding strain to your lower back.

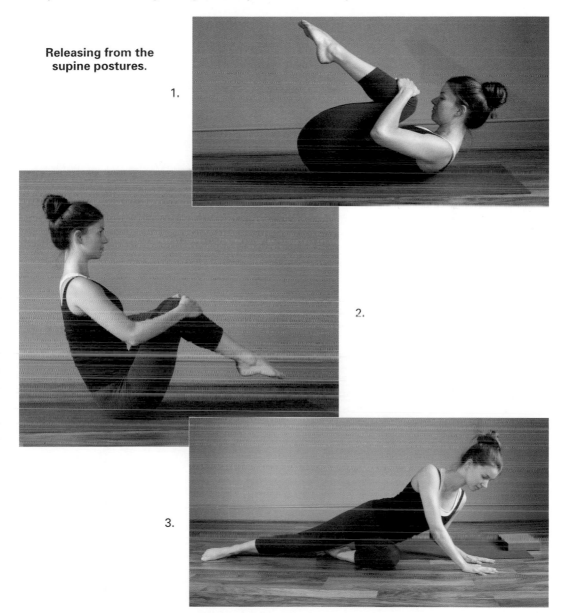

Releasing from the supine postures.

1.

2.

3.

3   Good Posture

It is a great asset to know how to hold your body with balance and ease. This is not only for maintaining good health – it also helps you feel confident. As we grow, it is easy to give way to faulty habits. This is particularly so in the modern world with mass technology and energy-saving devices which are designed to make our life 'easier'. Whether we are sitting, kneeling, standing, walking, or simply going about our daily work or play, it is important that we do not neglect our posture allowing ourselves to succumb to sloppy habits which can affect our body as we grow older. The 'faulty' positions become our comfort zones and if we are not careful, the resulting imbalances in our body can lead to strain in our muscles and joints. Bad backs, painful, stiff joints, muscular pains and digestive complaints are just some of the problems which made need medical attention as we get older, or at least compromise our ability to live life to the full.

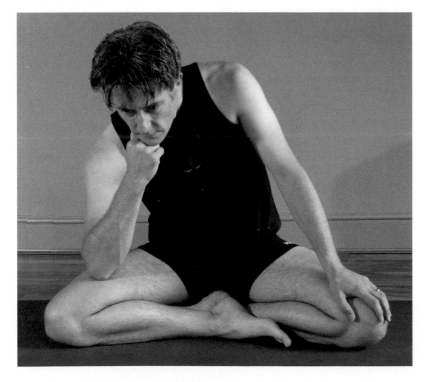

Here the spine is unnaturally curved, causing the back to 'hump'. The shoulders are rounded and the chest 'collapsed', causing restricted breathing. The weight of the body is unevenly distributed.

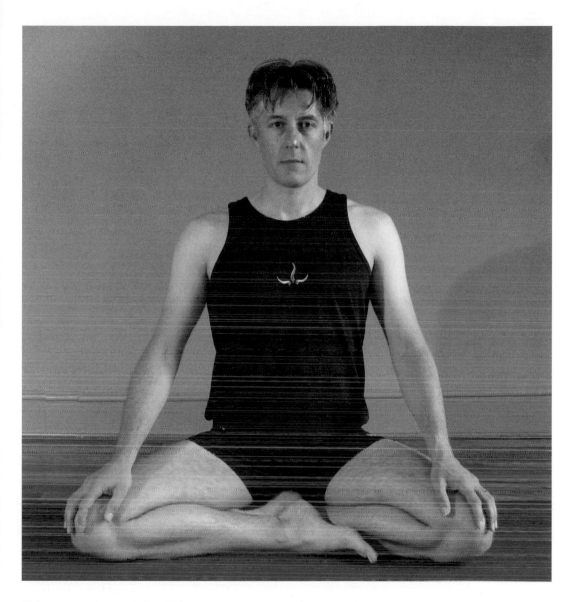

This posture is much healthier as well as being more pleasing
to look at. Note the air of confidence and ease.

Yoga is not about forcing our body into clever contortions. It is about bringing about awareness of how we are, physically and emotionally. With enhanced awareness comes the ability to recognize faulty patterns of functioning. Recognition is the key to correction and to the realization of our potential. The yoga postures may initially feel awkward and strange, but with regular practice they become easier and we develop new and healthier positions of 'comfort'.

What is good posture?

We can analyze posture by examining its components:

- The Foundation or Base. Whether we are lying, sitting, kneeling, standing, or inverted we need to feel stable and secure. The part of our body that is in contact with the ground is our foundation. The concept of being 'grounded' and 'down-to-earth' is about feeling stable and this is related to the earth's gravitational pull.
- Body Alignment and Dynamic. This is related to the way we 'hold' our body and provide resistance to the pull of gravity. A well-aligned body, based on an understanding of our skeletal and muscular systems, has balance and symmetry.
- Composure. It is essential that we are not distracted by feeling tense. There is limited benefit from stability and good alignment if we are agitated. The subtle component of posture is the ability to feel calm and stay focused. And it is this quality of being easy, that brings about the process of mind/body integration, transforming our practice from merely physical training into yoga.

We can apply the principles above to all our postures.

The Easy Pose

This is a way of sitting that is comfortable and 'easy'. It is a stable posture that was traditionally adopted for meditation. The broad base formed by the sitting bones of the pelvis, the legs and feet lends itself to good balance. Easy Pose involves crossing one leg over the other allowing the knees to roll out to the sides.

1. Sit on your mat on one or two blocks. The block(s) help to adjust the pelvis by tilting it to facilitate release of the spine. Focus on your pelvis and come onto the front of your sitting bones and towards the front of your block. Cross your legs, allowing your knees to roll out to the sides. Allow your knees and ankles to relax. Bring your attention to the contact of your sitting bones with the block and the sides of your feet with the mat. Adjust your position so that you feel balanced and stable.

2. Envisage the vertical rise of your trunk from your pelvis. Gently lift your sternum and roll your shoulders down and back so that your chest is full and broad. Your abdomen becomes longer and flatter with the lift of your rib cage. As you 'lengthen' the front of your body, your back will simultaneously extend allowing the vertical release of your spine. Let your arms rest comfortably by your sides and place your hands palms down on your knees. Bring your head into central balance at the top of your spine. Keep your chin tucked in slightly so that your throat is relaxed and the back of your neck assumes it natural length and curvature. The back of your head should lie in the same plane as your shoulder blades and back of your pelvis. Look directly ahead with your eyes open and focus soft.

Let go of inner tension – your composure can be enhanced by consciously relaxing your eyes, tongue root and lower jaw. This simple process to bring internal calm can be adopted in all postures. Now focus on your breath and the sensations in your body as you hold the posture.

Modification: unless your back is reasonably strong, you may find the above way of sitting uncomfortable, in which case it helps to sit with your back against a wall. This will provide you with firm support until you are ready to sit unaided. Place your block(s) against a wall and sit on them so that the back of your pelvis makes contact with the skirting board and the back of your body and head are supported by the wall.

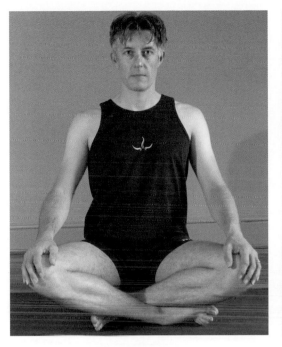

The Easy Pose.

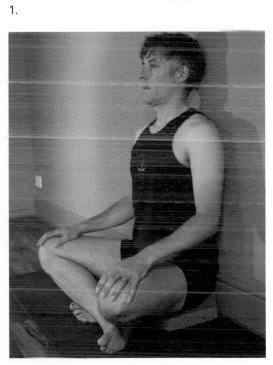

1.

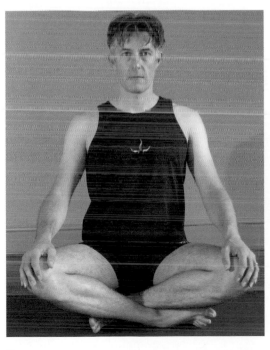

2.

Modification.

The Adepts Pose

Adept (meaning 'skilled') is a very stable way of sitting, which requires a moderate degree of flexibility in the pelvic joints. It is a classical pose for meditation.

1. Sit on your block(s) with legs straight. Move onto the front of your sitting bones and towards the front of the block. Bend your right knee and bring your heel close into your groin. Take your bent knee down to mat.
2. Bend your left leg and place the heel of your left foot so that it rests in front of and in contact with your right heel and ankle. Allow your left knee to rest on the mat.
3. Having established your foundation, proceed as in Easy Pose bringing alignment and symmetry to your posture whilst relaxing your eyes, tongue root and lower jaw to maintain inner calm.

Caution: it is important that you do not feel strain in your pelvic joints and that your knees rest comfortably on the mat. If you are having difficulties in the posture, keep with Easy Pose until you develop greater flexibility in your pelvic joints.

Modification: if you cannot get your knees to rest comfortably on the mat, sitting on two blocks might make it easier. If necessary, use the modification described for Easy Pose, sitting with your back against a wall for added support. You may find that both Easy Pose and Adepts Pose are uncomfortable, in which case it may be better for you to sit with your legs straight out. Be prepared to try different positions at this stage. It is important that you are comfortable and stable.

In both Easy Pose and Adepts Pose, remember to alternate the position of your legs. In other words, if you are sitting for some time with right leg in front of left, reverse the legs so that left rests in front of right for an equivalent time. This is to maintain balance and to avoid getting into a comfort zone favouring one leg arrangement over the other.

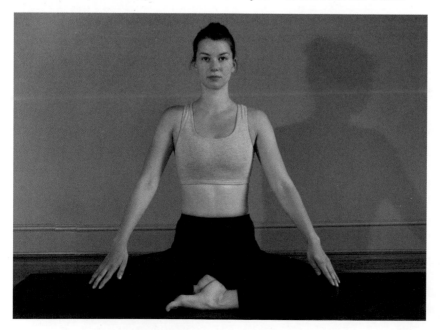

The Adepts Pose.

The Seated Stretch

This is an excellent way of awakening your body by lengthening your trunk and releasing your spine.

1. Sit in Easy Pose or Adepts Pose (or with your legs straight out). Bring your arms in front of you, palms facing in. Open your palms and spread your fingers. Keep your sternum up and engaging the muscles of your arms, observe the charge of energy from shoulders to elbows, elbows to wrists and into your fingertips. Take two or three breaths.

2. Inhaling, raise your arms pointing your fingertips towards the ceiling. Push your fingers gently upwards whilst keeping your pelvis firmly down on the block. Avoid lifting your shoulders – move them downwards away from your ears. As you reach up feel the lift of your ribcage causing your abdomen to lengthen and flatten. At the same time, observe how your back lengthens allowing the release of your spine. Take two to three breaths.

The Seated Stretch.

1.

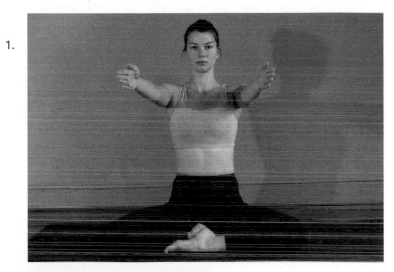

2.

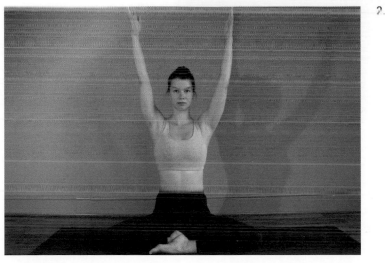

3. Clasp your fingers, put the tips of your thumbs together and turning your palms upwards, push them towards the ceiling increasing the intensity of the stretch. Take two to three breaths before changing the clasp and pushing your palms up again. Be prepared to bring challenge to your stretch whilst taking care not to strain. Breathe freely, maintaining internal calm.

4. To release, exhale as you return your hands to your knees.

3.

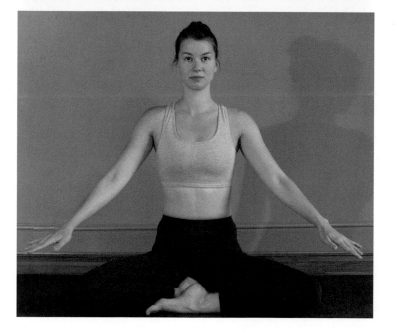

4.

Coming out of Easy Pose and Adepts Pose

When sitting with legs crossed for some time you may find that your knees and ankles get a bit stiff. If you are sitting on two blocks, come down onto one. Extend your legs and push your toes away from you, engaging your leg muscles and gently opening the backs of your knees (see Fig. 1). Now bring your toes towards you pushing into your heels (see Fig. 2). Maintain a rhythm of flexing and extending your feet for several repetitions. The squeezing effect on the leg muscles helps to stimulate the venous blood flow and you will feel the release of any stiffness in your knees and ankles.

The Leg Stretch.

1.

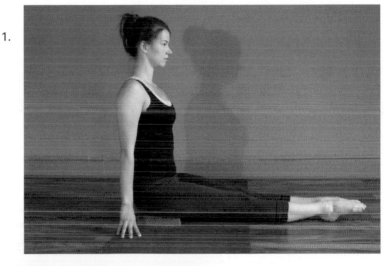

2.

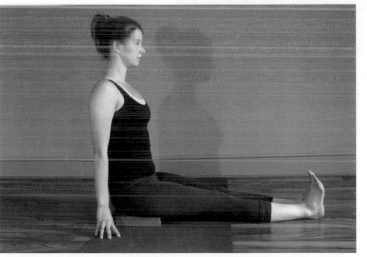

Playing the edge

Whilst working in postures it is important that we control our movements to avoid over-stretching and exceeding our limit and it is essential that we exercise appropriate caution so that we do not put adverse strain on our body which could result in injury. On the other hand, it is necessary that we feel free and are willing to challenge ourselves enough to promote activity that will take us into new territory and make us feel good. Yoga is a subtle art and science which involves continually adjusting our movements to find balance. This process of discovering that fine line of caution on the one hand and adventure on the other is about 'playing the edge'. Like life itself, perhaps?

As your yoga skills develop, so your 'edge' will change as you become fitter, stronger and more flexible. And this – together with your ability to remain focused – will give you a greater zest for life and an increased confidence. But do have patience and resist the temptation to push ahead too quickly, risking strain or injury.

The Hero Pose
This pose (hero: a man of noble qualities) is a kneeling posture, which involves sitting on the heels whilst holding the body still and erect.

1. Come up onto your knees with feet apart and arms extending by your sides.
2. Put your big toes together, let your heels separate and prepare to sit on your heels. As you sit, pull your calf muscles out to the sides before resting your pelvis on your heels.
3. Place your hands palms down and with fingers gently open, onto your knees and take time to establish your base, allowing your pelvis, knees, ankles and feet to relax.
4. Bring alignment and symmetry into your posture. Gently lift your sternum allowing your abdomen to lengthen and

flatten. Feel the extension of your back and the release of your spine. Bring your head into central balance and roll your shoulders down and back so that your chest is full and broad. Allow your eyes, tongue root and lower jaw to soften to help bring inner calm. Breathe freely and look straight ahead with your eyes open and your focus soft.

Caution: this posture does not suit everyone, particularly if there is stiffness in the knees and ankles. Be wary of your knee joints, taking care not to cause overstretch. Use the modifications below if they help, or come out of the posture if it does not feel right.

Modifications: if you have difficulty sitting on your heels, this may be due to stiffness in your knee joints. In which case, place a block(s) or folded blanket on your heels and make sure your pelvis is fully supported. Also, if the tops of your feet or ankles are uncomfortable, place a folded blanket under your feet.

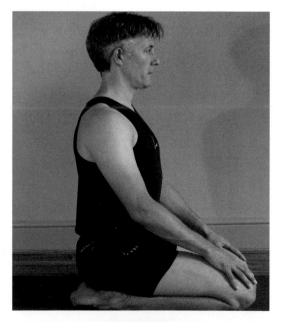

The Hero Pose.

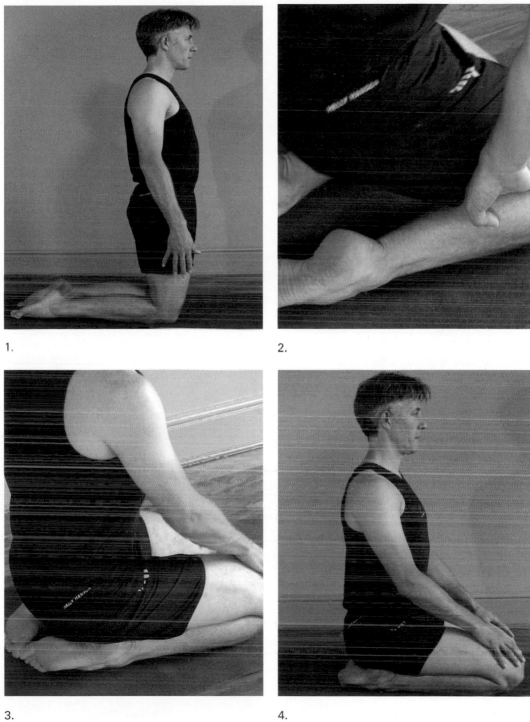

1.

2.

3.

4.

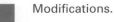

Modifications.

The Hero Stretch

This stretch awakens the trunk and spine.

1. Clasp your fingers, place the tips of your thumbs together and push your palms away from you. Feel the charge of energy in your arms. Keep your sternum up and breathe freely. Change the clasp and push again.
2. Inhale as you push your palms to the ceiling whilst keeping your pelvis firmly down and breathe freely as you stretch your trunk. You will feel your rib cage lift and your abdomen lengthen and flatten. The extension of your back will allow the release of your spine. Feel the energy in your trunk as you stretch. Change the clasp and push your palms up again, focusing on the sensations in your body. Exhale as you release, returning your hands to your knees to settle back into Hero Pose.

Modification: as described for Hero Pose.

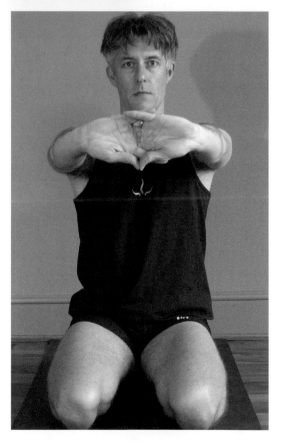

The Hero Stretch. 1.

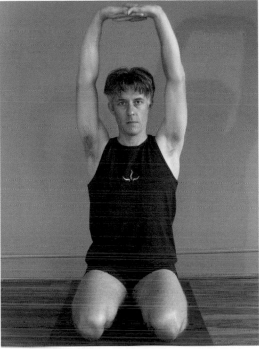

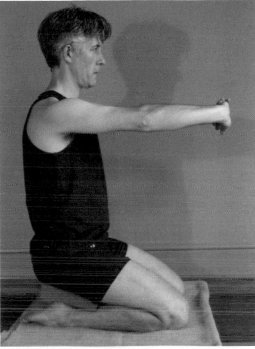

2.   Modifications.

Spiralling

In his book, *Dynamic Yoga*, Godfrey Devereux[3] states that the way we use our limbs to support the foundation in our postures is crucial. He adeptly explains how the muscles are used to cradle and support the bones to make them stable and that this involves lengthening and sealing muscle groups into the bone. He describes the experience of the sealing process as 'a sucking sensation of the muscles into the bone'. Devereux discusses the mechanism of the spiral, which is a subtle way of turning the limbs in such a way as to rotate the muscles in opposing directions, similar to the action of twisting the fibres of a rope to make it stronger.

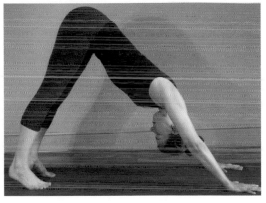

The Down Facing Dog Pose.

The Down Facing Dog Pose
This classical yoga posture resembles the stretch of a dog as it rouses itself from sleep. It is an excellent posture for stretching the back and spine and the legs. Regular practice will strengthen and energize the whole body.

1. Come up onto your hands and knees (the 'all-fours' position). The hands, knees and tops of feet provide the stable base. With the hands at shoulder width, open your palms and spread your fingers, middle fingers pointing forwards. Push your palms firmly into the mat. Look back at your knees, which need to be at hip width, with your thighs vertical. Rest on the tops of your feet keeping them at the same distance apart as your knees. Feel your support on the mat, making sure that you are evenly balanced. Keep your head and neck relaxed and direct your gaze downwards.
2. In Down Facing Dog Pose we spiral the arms. Keep your hands stable, your arms straight and rotate your upper arms so that your biceps face forwards. As the arms extend out of the wrists the lower arms turn inwards whilst the upper arms rotate outwards with opposition at the elbow joints. This gives the arms strength and stability.
3. To move into the full posture, tuck your toes under and lifting onto the balls of your feet, push you pelvis backwards and upwards allowing your legs to straighten. You will feel your trunk and spine lengthen as you push your pelvis away and tilt it towards the ceiling. As the distance between your pelvis and rib cage increases your abdomen will become longer and flatter. Draw in your navel and keep your armpits up with your

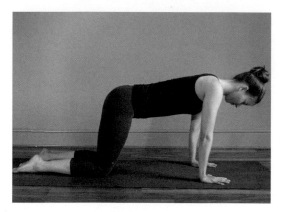

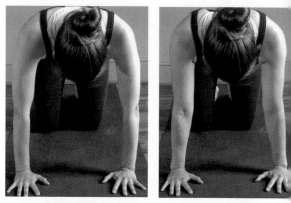

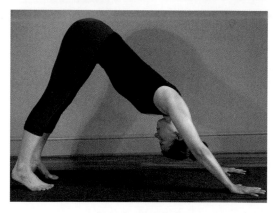

CLOCKWISE FROM TOP LEFT:

1. 'All fours' position.

2(i). Neutral position.

2(ii). Spiral the arms.

3. Full posture.

chest broad, shoulder blades pressing into your back. Gently push your heels down towards the mat taking care not to hyperextend the backs of your knees or to overstretch your hamstrings. Release your head and look back at your feet and ankles with face relaxed. Breathe freely and with full awareness maintaining internal calm.

Caution: take care not to hyperextend the backs of your knees or to overstretch your hamstrings. The hamstrings are a group of tendons at the back of the knee and attached to the tibia below. Athletes and the elderly are especially prone to tight hamstrings. Tilting the pelvis upwards and backwards causes the hamstrings to lengthen and care must be taken to avoid overstretching them. Resist the temptation to compromise your spinal stretch in your attempt to fully straighten your legs. If your hamstrings are tight, there is the probability that you would round and flatten your back and prevent full release of your spine (see A, below). In which case, you will need to bend your knees slightly so that you can achieve the full spinal stretch whilst at the same time protecting your hamstrings (see B, below). With practice your hamstrings should become less tight, making it easier for you to open the backs of your knees and straighten your legs.

Protecting the hamstrings.

A. Incorrect.

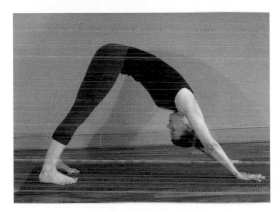

B. Correct.

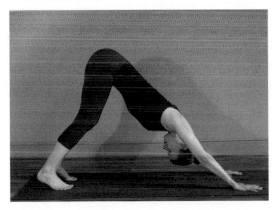

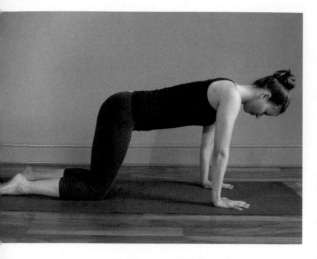

Release to 'all-fours'.

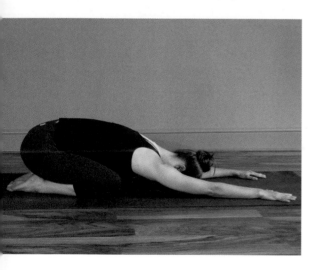

Release to Down Facing Hero Pose.

Keeping postures dynamic

Keeping our postures lively during the 'holding' stage requires continual small and subtle adjustments in order to maintain balance, to avoid strain and discomfort and to invite challenge. It is by being mindful to what we are experiencing moment by moment that enables us to find our edge and gain maximum benefit from our postures. As we progress in our yoga our body develops an 'understanding' which helps to guide us into our optimum pose. The enhanced sensitivity which evolves with practice helps us to finely tune our postures so that they remain dynamic, rather than becoming static and boring.

Maintaining the dynamic in Down Facing Dog Pose

Gently push the backs of your knees away from your trunk whilst moving your chest towards the fronts of your knees. Keep your armpits up and your chest broad, pressing your shoulder blades into your back. Hold your navel in towards your spine. Observe the lines of energy in your body, one passing upwards from the crown of your head, along your spine and pelvis towards the ceiling, another passing downwards from the back of your pelvis, along your legs, into your heels and towards the mat. Breathe deeply and freely with your face relaxed and give your full attention to the sensations in your body and to your breath.

Releasing from Down Facing Dog Pose

To release, return to your hands and knees. Allow your back to settle by moving into the Down Facing Hero Pose, which is the next posture to be described.

The Down Facing Hero Pose

This allows the lower back to settle whilst maintaining a gentle stretch on the spine and trunk. It brings steadiness to the mind and body.

1. Commence in the all-fours position. Place your big toes together and separate your heels.
2. Push your pelvis downwards and backwards onto your heels. Maintain a stretch in your arms with palms open and fingers spread. Release your head so that your forehead rests comfortably on the mat and allow your face and forehead to relax. Keep your arms straight, your armpits up and your chest broad. Hold the posture and breathe freely, observing the gentle stretch of your back and spine.

**The Down Facing
Hero Pose.**

1.

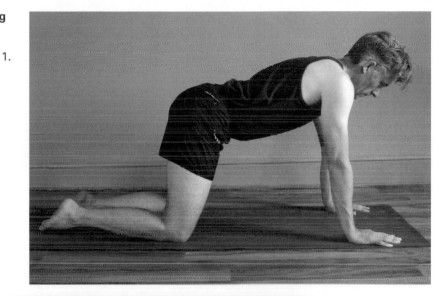

2.

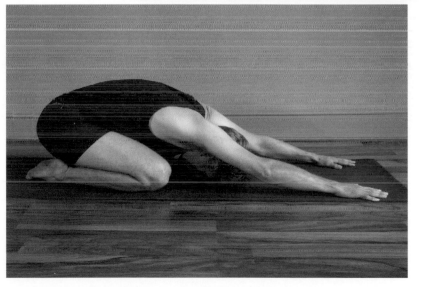

3. To release, walk your hands back to your knees and, lifting your head and trunk, return to Hero Pose.

Modification: if your forehead does not rest comfortably on the mat, then support it with a block or blocks. It is important you do not put strain on your neck. If your pelvis does not sit comfortably on your heels, place a folded blanket or block(s) on your heels to give your pelvis support. If necessary, rest your feet and ankles on a folded blanket.

Caution: avoid strain in your knee joints by ensuring that your pelvis is fully supported.

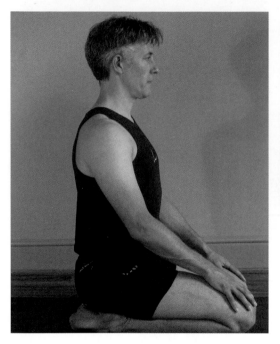

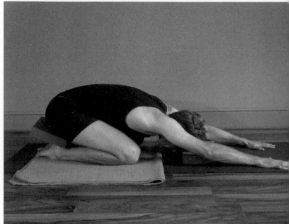

LEFT: 3.

ABOVE: Modification.

Holding in yoga postures

There is no standard length of time you should stay in your posture. In the early stages of your practice you may find that some of the postures feel strange and uncomfortable. This is inevitable while you are learning new techniques and developing different ways of using your body. You are moving beyond your comfort zones and you may find that you soon feel strain. In the early stages of practice it is wise to be cautious, holding the postures for a short time only, say three to four breaths. As you become fitter and more adept you will want to gradually extend the holding period. A good guide is to stay in the posture as long as you feel the process is doing you good and come out if you experience strain or discomfort. As the 'intelligence' in your body develops you will come to know the stage at which you should release.

The three stages
There are three stages to each posture: entering, holding and the release. It is important that you undertake each stage with care and full attention. At all times be mindful of your breath and the sensations in your body.

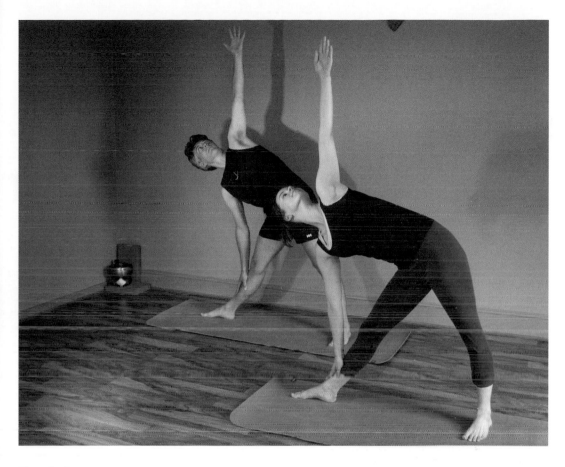

Yoga in harmony.

Balanced energy

Yoga is aptly qualified as relaxation in action. This cleverly emphasizes how the practice of yoga postures creates balanced energy. Excessive action will cause our energy to dissipate, whilst too little leads to stagnation. We learn to bring balance to the opposing forces of action and receptivity. Too much emphasis on one or the other creates disharmony.

4　The Standing Postures

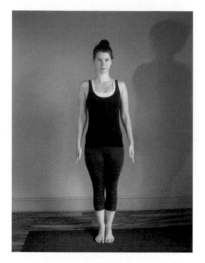

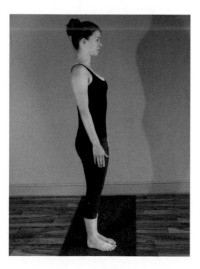

The Mountain Pose.

The standing postures promote good balance, alignment, strength and flexibility. They are generally enlivening and regular practice brings steadiness and grace. All standing postures have the feet as their foundation. They are energizing postures and although they can be practised at any time, they are especially beneficial in the early part of the day when we need energy for the days' activities.

The Mountain Pose
We contemplate the mountain as still, stable, strong and silent and this aptly describes the posture.

1. Stand on the mat with your feet together, making contact with your big toes and ankles. Lift onto the balls of your feet and stretch your heels back before settling them on the mat. Lift your toes and spread them wide and maintain the spread as you settle them down. Feel the soles of your feet on the mat and rock gently back and forth before returning to balance. Now gently rotate on your feet, bringing your attention to outer edges and balls of feet, inner edges and heels. Rotate in the opposite direction before settling into good balance.
2. Bring awareness to your legs. Engage your thigh muscles, applying the concept of the sucking sensation of the muscles into the bones. As you engage your thigh

muscles, the backs of your knees will open and your knee caps will engage. Take care not to hyperextend the backs of your knees by pushing them back too hard. Now, shift attention to your pelvis. Clenching your buttocks, lengthen your tail bone (coccyx). This will help stabilize your pelvis, which is necessary for maintaining the integrity of the spine.

Caution: it is important to avoid the problem of exaggerating the lumbar curve in the lower back. This occurs when the pelvis tilts excessively backwards so that the tail bone sticks out. This can result in back strain. Pelvic stability is maintained by keeping the tail bone 'long' thus maintaining the natural curvature in the lumbar spine.

3. The legs and pelvis support the upper body. Lift your sternum allowing your abdomen to lengthen and flatten. (The lengthening of the abdomen brings tone to the abdominal muscles. A well-toned abdomen provides support to the lower back.) Release your shoulders, moving them down away from your ears, and roll them back allowing your chest to become full, broad and active. Extend your arms by your sides with your palms facing in and fingers lightly spread. Bring your head into central balance. The back of your head should be in line with the back of your shoulder blades and pelvis. Look straight ahead with your eyes open and your focus soft. Relax your eyes, tongue root and lower jaw and take a few moments to establish your inner calm. Breathe freely and hold the posture with full awareness focusing on your breath and on the sensations in your body.

Modification: If you feel unstable, stand with your back against a wall. This will provide you with support so that you feel

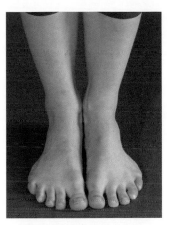

1. Feet as the foundation.

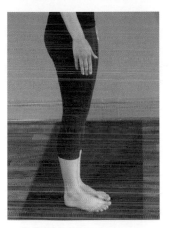

2. Legs and pelvis.

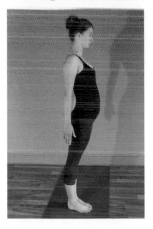

Incorrect alignment.

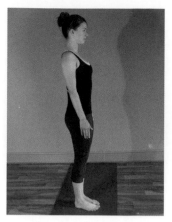

Correct alignment.

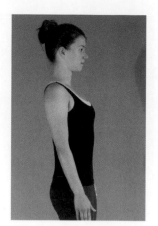

3. Upper body.

stable. It will also help your body alignment. Keep your heels, pelvis, shoulder blades and back of your head in contact with the wall.

The Standing Stretch
An excellent way of extending the body, energizing the trunk and releasing the spine.

1. Commence in Mountain Pose. Inhaling, raise your arms above your head. Open your palms and push your fingertips towards the ceiling. Do not lift your shoulders. Keep them down away from your ears so that your neck is long and free from tension. As you push your fingers up to the ceiling, press the soles of your feet firmly into the mat, keeping your thigh muscles engaged and your tailbone long to maintain pelvic stability. Observe the lift of your rib cage and the lengthening of your abdomen. As your back extends you will feel the release of your spine. Breathe freely and hold the stretch with full awareness and inner calm.

2. Clasp your fingers, place the tips of your thumbs together and turning your palms upwards, push them towards the ceiling, gently increasing the stretch. Keep the downward momentum by pressing the

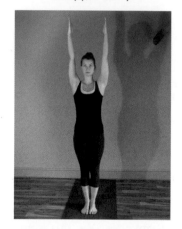

The Standing Stretch. 1. Correct.

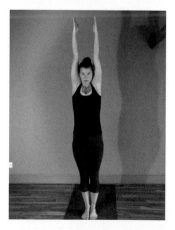

Incorrect.

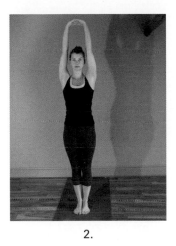

2.

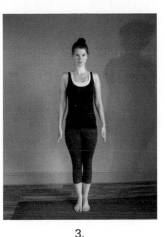

3.

soles of your feet firmly into the mat, with legs strong and pelvis stable. After two or three breaths, change the clasp, push up again and hold the stretch, breathing freely with full awareness and inner calm.

3. To release, exhale as you bring your arms to your sides, returning to Mountain Pose.

Extending from the core

We think of the centre of our body as our 'core'. When we talk about core strength, we tend associate this with the power in our abdominal muscles. Yet this central region located around our navel is also related to our solar plexus, which is a complex of nerves and an energy centre at the pit of the stomach. As we extend our body as for example in the Standing Stretch, we are in effect directing our energy so that it expands and extends from our centre towards our periphery. With each inhalation our energy is channelled to infiltrate every part of our body. The reverse is true as we exhale: by the technique of 'letting go' we allow our energy to flow back to our centre or core. This regular process of action and release to coincide with inhaling and exhaling helps to build our strength and vitality but at the same time keeps us feeling free and relaxed. This rein-

forces the idea of yoga as relaxation in action. By establishing the concept of our core as our centre of energy and by understanding the process of energy flow, we come to regard our body as a whole rather than a collection of parts. In the Standing Stretch there are two main lines of energy extending from the core: upwards towards the fingertips and downwards towards the soles of the feet.

The shoulders

It is not uncommon to hold tension in the shoulders. This happens when we are feeling stressed and tired. Rounding or hunching of the shoulders is a sign of prolonged tension.

The Shoulder Roll

A simple exercise to release tension in the shoulders.

1. Commence in Mountain Pose. Lift your shoulders towards your ears, then roll them backwards and downwards feeling your shoulder blades press into your back. Repeat this rolling movement several times, paying particular attention to the sensations in your shoulder girdle.

2. Reverse the movement, rolling your shoulders in the opposite direction.

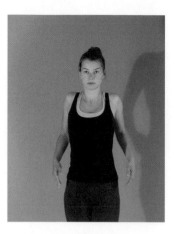

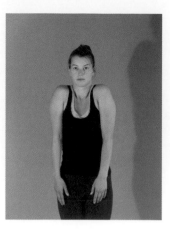

The Shoulder Roll. 1.

2.

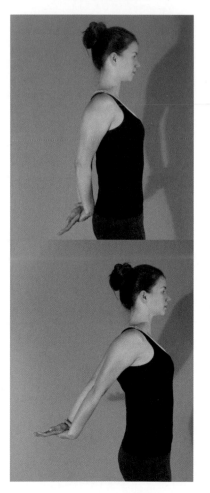

The Shoulder Stretch

This releases tension in the shoulder joints and helps correct the tendency to round shoulders.

1. Commence in Mountain Pose. Take your arms behind you and clasp your right wrist firmly with your left hand.
2. Straighten your arms and pull them away from your back. As you do this you will feel your chest broaden and your shoulder blades press into your back. Keep your pelvis stable with your tail bone long so that you do not exaggerate the curve in your lower back. Release and clasping the opposite wrist, repeat the movement.

The Shoulder Stretch.

TOP LEFT: 1.

LEFT: 2.

Standing balances

It is known that our sense of balance deteriorates as we get older. The next two postures involve standing on one leg and are useful in developing and maintaining good balance. They also exercise the leg muscles and strengthen the ankles as well as promoting mental calm.

The Crane Pose

The crane is a large wading bird with long legs. It is seen standing on one leg for long periods in shallow water.

1. Commence in Mountain Pose. Rest your hands on your hips and keep your pelvis stable. Take your weight onto your right foot and raise your left knee pointing your toes downwards. Keep your right leg straight and firm but take care not to hyperextend the back of your knee. Hold the posture for several breaths keeping your pelvis stable with tail bone long, your chest up and shoulders rolling gently down and back. With head in central balance look straight ahead with eyes open and focus soft and maintain inner calm. It is especially important in standing balances to pay full attention to the sensations in your body and to your breath. This helps to keep the mind steady and helps prevent loss of balance. Release and repeat on the opposite side, this time keeping your left leg straight and raising your right knee.

Modification: if you have difficulty balancing then stand with your back either against the wall or at right angles to the wall (see overleaf). This will provide support and give you confidence whilst you are developing your technique.

Caution: if you are at all uncertain about your balancing ability, then use the wall as support until you are more confident.

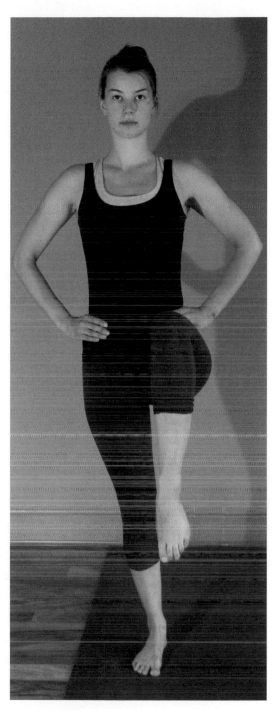

The Crane Pose

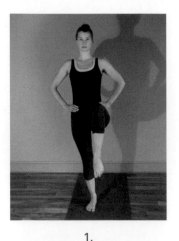

1.

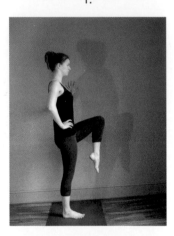

Modification.

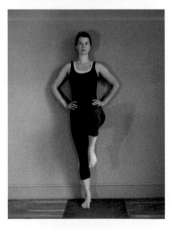

Modification.

Note: in many of the postures especially where you are balancing on one leg, you may find that you have a 'good side' where the posture feels more comfortable and a 'not so good side' which is less stable. It is important that you do not neglect your less comfortable side. In fact, there is a case for practising more on your difficult side until both sides become equally comfortable. You will have noticed a pattern in posture work: whatever action you do on one side of the body, you repeat on the opposite side. It is necessary to maintain symmetry and balance.

The Tree Pose

This symbolizes both physical and spiritual life. The roots take nourishment from the earth and keep the tree stable, whilst the branches reach to the heavens in exaltation. The posture develops strength and composure and improves flexibility in the pelvis.

1. Commence in Mountain Pose. Place your hands on your hips to stabilize your pelvis and shift your weight onto your left foot.
2. Take hold of your right ankle and bring your right heel up to your groin placing the sole of the foot against your left inner thigh, toes pointing downwards. Roll your right knee out to the side whilst keeping your pelvis facing squarely forwards. Take a few moments to find your balance. As you take the weight onto your left foot and raise your right heel, there will be a subtle shift in your centre of gravity. This will require a slight movement of your body to the left to compensate.
3. Extend your arms out to the sides to assist your stability.
4. Inhaling, raise your arms above your head, pointing your fingers to the ceiling, palms facing in. Do not lift your shoulders – move them down away from your ears. Keep your chest up, abdomen

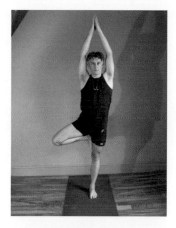

The Tree Pose.

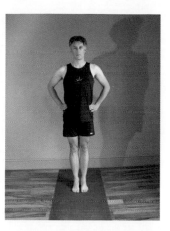

1.

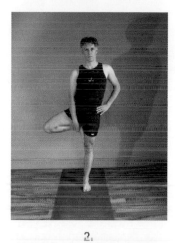

2.

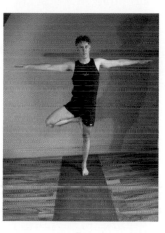

3.

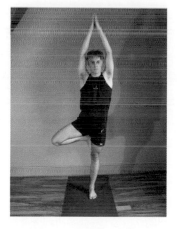

4.

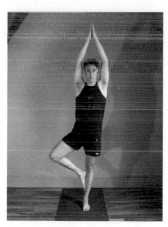

Modification.

long and your pelvis stable. Your straight leg should be strong and firm but take care not to hyperextend the back of your knee. With head in central balance, keep your eyes open, your focus soft and maintain inner calm. Breathe freely and hold the pose for several breaths. (Note: it may help your balance if you focus on a fixed point at eye level on the wall in front of you.)

Modification: if you have difficulty balancing, stand with your back against a wall or stand at right angles to the wall. If you have difficulty lifting your heel into the groin, then rest your foot further down your leg.

Caution: if you are at all uncertain about your balancing ability then use the wall for support until you feel more confident.

The next group of standing postures has the advantage of a stable foundation which is accomplished by taking the feet into a wide stride. By keeping the legs strong and the pelvis stable, you are providing the firm base from which you can exercise your upper body, bringing suppleness to the trunk and spine.

The Extended Triangle Pose
This pose provides a strong, side stretch.

1. Commence in Mountain Pose. Take a wide stride of approximately one metre. Keep your feet parallel and your toes in line (a good guide is to have your toes parallel with the front of the mat). Rest your hands on your hips and ensure that you are evenly balanced on both feet. Engage your thigh muscles taking care not to hyperextend the backs of your knees. Keep your tail bone long and stabilize your pelvis. Lift your sternum and roll your shoulders down and back so

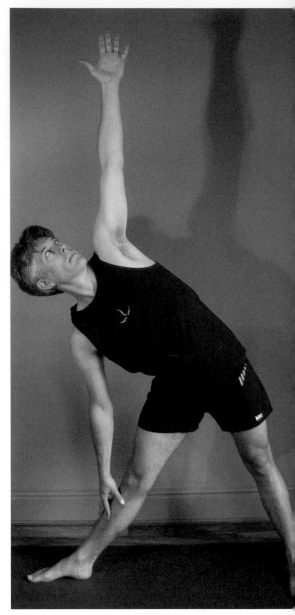

The Extended Triangle Pose.

that your chest is full and broad, your abdomen long and flat. Bring your head into central balance and look directly ahead.

2. Rotate on your left heel turning your left foot inwards at an angle of approximately ten to fifteen degrees. Lift onto your right heel and rotate your right foot through ninety degrees rolling your right knee and thigh in the same outwards direction. The heel of your right foot should be in line with the inner arch of your left foot. You may find that your pelvis and trunk have turned slightly to the right. In which case, roll back your left hip and left shoulder so that your pelvis and trunk face squarely forwards.

3. Inhaling, raise your arms taking them into the "T" position and keep your chest up. Spread your palms and lengthen into your fingertips. Turn your palms up to the ceiling and then rotate your hands so that your palms face downwards. This will bring about the process of spiralling of the arms (see below).

4. Turn the outer edge of your left foot firmly in towards the mat. This will keep your left leg strong as you prepare to extend your trunk to the right (this process of providing resistance is described in greater detail below). Extend your trunk to the right keeping both sides of your torso of equal length. Roll your left arm behind you and keep your left shoulder and left hip rolling back so that your pelvis and trunk stay facing squarely forwards.

5. Take your right fingertips down onto your right shin taking care not to overstretch. Your legs, pelvis, trunk and head should lie in the same plane as if your whole body were between two panes of glass.

6. Look over your left shoulder and, inhaling, raise your left arm, palm facing forwards and direct your gaze to your left

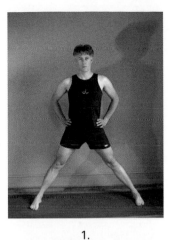

1.

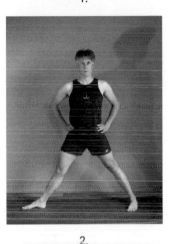

2.

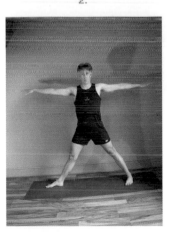

3.

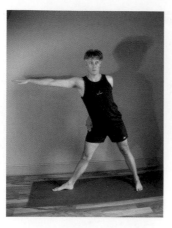

4.

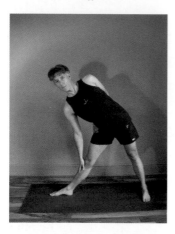

5.

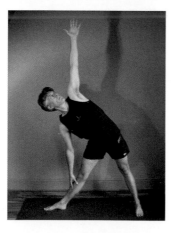

6.

thumb. Hold the posture without strain for three to four breaths paying full attention to the sensations in your body. Maintain inner calm.

To release from extended triangle, inhale and maintaining the resistance on your left side, return to upright. Exhaling, release your arms, returning your hands to your hips and bring your feet back to parallel. Repeat on the opposite side before returning to Mountain Pose.

Caution: do not overstretch as this will spoil the posture and place unnecessary strain on the body. In Fig. B opposite, note the loss of alignment due to overstretch. It is important to keep your legs, pelvis, trunk, head and arms in the same plane (Fig. A, opposite). Always keep the stretch within your limit, focusing on the quality rather than the quantity of the movement. Also, ensure that your neck is relaxed as you direct your gaze to your top thumb.

Modification: if you find difficulty with stability and alignment, practice the posture with the back of your body against a wall until you become more adept.

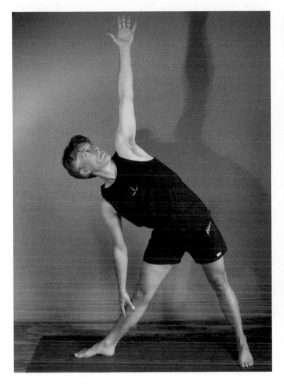

A. Correct alignment.

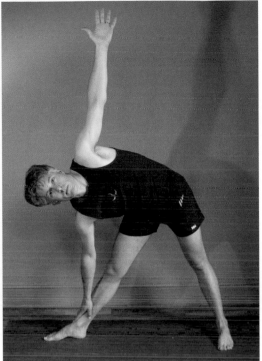

B. Incorrect due to over-stretching.

Resistance

When we are standing there is a gravitational pull on our body which keeps our feet on the ground. It is the resistance to the pull of gravity that keeps us upright. Muscular effort is required to maintain this resistance and it is this effort that produces muscular tone. If our muscles are weak our ability to resist the gravitational pull on our body is affected and our posture suffers. As we move our body in performing various yoga postures, our centre of gravity changes and to avoid adverse strain as we move our body to change our position, we need to provide resistance by making subtle counter adjustments in order to maintain body balance. In the case of Extended Triangle, as we move our body in one direction we apply resistance in the opposite direction.

In Extended Triangle as we extend our body to the right we need to provide resistance on the left. By turning the outer side of the left foot firmly into the mat, whilst slightly lifting the inner arch, the left leg is kept strong thereby distributing the load more evenly as we extend the trunk to the right. Without resistance, the right leg would have to support most of the body's weight, resulting in imbalance.

Spiralling the arms
The mechanism of The Spiral has already been discussed in relation to Down Facing Dog Pose. Godfrey Devereux[4] elucidates the principle of the spiral in standing postures. He affirms that by creating a spirallic momentum, full power and maximum stability are given to the limbs. In Extended

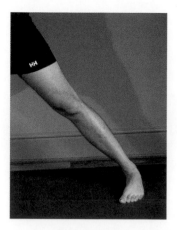

Resistance.

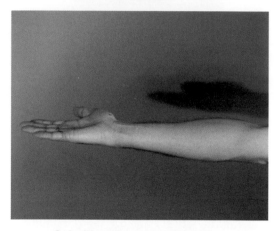

Spiralling the arms. Palms up.

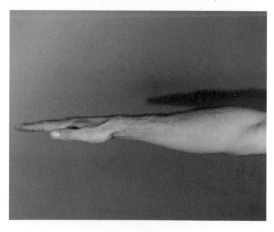

Palms down.

Triangle the arms are raised into the 'T' position. By extending the arms as far out from the shoulders as possible and by spreading the palms carrying the extension from the wrists into the fingertips, the arms become longer and stronger as the muscles 'suck' into the bone. The spirallic momentum is fully effected by turning the palms up to the ceiling then rotating them downwards to face the floor so that muscle groups in the arms are in opposition. (As the wrists and lower arms rotate inwards the biceps in the upper arms remain upwards with opposition at the elbow joint.) The 'twisting', together with the lengthening, bring strength and stability to the arms, which become highly energized. Devereux likens this to the effect of twisting the fibres of a rope to give it maximum strength.

The Side Warrior Pose

The Warrior Poses are symbolic of the ancient, distinguished and experienced soldier. The postures develop steadiness, strength and physical and mental control. (There are three Warrior Poses, two of which are covered here.)

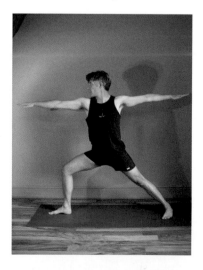

The Side Warrior Pose.

1. Commence in Mountain Pose. Take a wide stride of approximately one metre, feet parallel and toes in line. Engage your thigh muscles and stabilize your pelvis keeping your tail bone long. Lift your sternum and release your shoulders, moving them down and back so that your chest is full, broad and active, and your abdomen is long and flat. Bring your head into central balance and rest your hands on your hips.

2. Rotate on your left heel, turning your left foot in at an angle of ten to fifteen degrees. Lift onto your right heel and rotate your right foot through ninety degrees rolling your right knee and thigh in the same outward direction. The heel of your right foot should be in line with the inner arch of your left foot. Adjust your pelvis and trunk to face squarely forwards. Inhaling, take your arms out into the 'T' position. Spread your palms and extend into your fingertips. Turn your palms up to the ceiling then spiral your arms by rotating your palms to face downwards. Create resistance in your left leg by turning the outer side of your left foot firmly in towards the mat.

3. Bend your right knee until it rests directly above your heel and ankle. Ensure that your trunk stays vertical and does not lean. This can be helped by 'pulling back' along your left arm to create resistance.

4. Turn your head to the right and look over your right shoulder, directing your gaze along your right arm and right, middle finger. Breathe freely and hold the posture with full awareness and inner calm.

5. To release, inhale as you carefully straighten your right knee whilst maintaining resistance on your left side. Exhale, as you return your hands to your hips and your feet to parallel. Repeat on opposite side before returning to Mountain Pose.

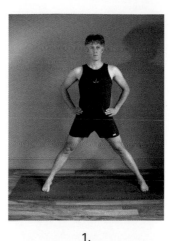

1.

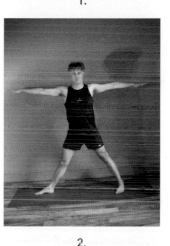

2.

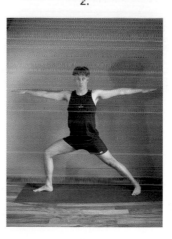

3.

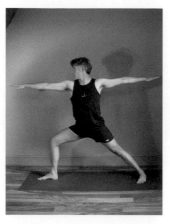

4.

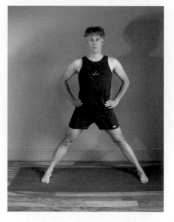

5.

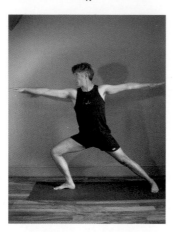

Problems associated with the Side Warrior Pose.

Bending too far. 6.

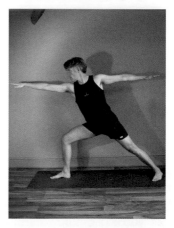

Knee rolling in. 7.

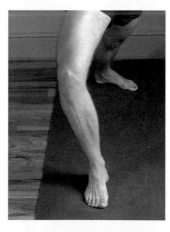

Knee rolling out. 8.

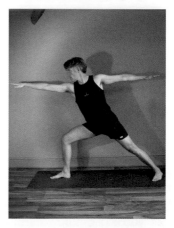

The trunk is leaning to the right. 9.

Caution: the relationship of the knee to the ankle and heel is of vital importance. To avoid strain or injury to the knee joint, the knee must rest directly over and above the heel and ankle. If we bend too far (see Fig. 6, previous page) the knee is unsupported. Support will also be lost if the knee rolls inwards or outwards (see Figs. 7 and 8). Ideally, when the knee is directly over the heel and ankle, the thigh should be parallel to the mat with the angle between thigh and shin bone at ninety degrees. However, this will depend on having a wide initial stride. Avoid 'leaning' (see Fig 9). 'Pulling back' along the left arm provides resistance to leaning.

The Warrior Pose

1. Commence in Mountain Pose. Take a wide stride of approximately one metre with feet parallel and toes in line.
2. Take your hands to your hips and turn your trunk to the right through an angle of ninety degrees so that your right foot faces forwards and your left foot rotates through an angle of around sixty degrees. Adjust your feet so that your front heel is in line with your back ankle. Bring the left side of your pelvis round so that your pelvis faces squarely forwards over your front leg. Engage your thigh muscles and stabilize your pelvis keeping your tail bone long. Keep your sternum up, your abdomen long and flat and your head in central balance.
3. Bend your front knee until your knee rests directly over your heel and ankle. Provide resistance by keeping your back thigh muscle engaged as you bend your front knee. Place your hands in front of your chest with palms together, fingers pointing upwards. Keep your trunk vertical (do not lean forwards).
4. Inhale as you raise your arms, pushing your fingers up towards the ceiling. As

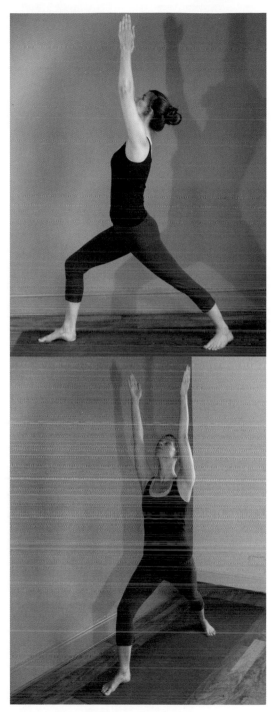

The Warrior Pose.

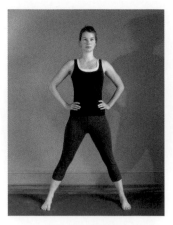

1.

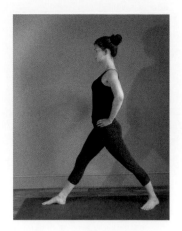

2.

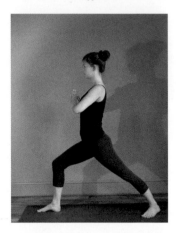

3.

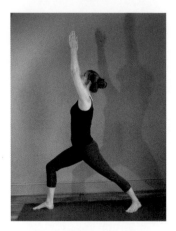

4.

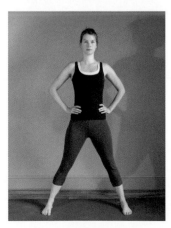

5.

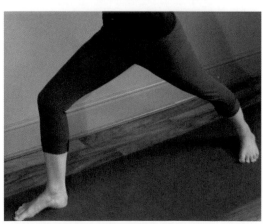

Turn the back foot through sixty degrees.

you raise your arms, feel your rib cage lift, your abdomen lengthen and flatten and your spine release. Separate your palms and look up. Maintain the resistance in your back leg muscles. Breathe freely with full awareness of the sensations in your body. Maintain inner calm.

5. To release, exhale as your return your hands to your hips and carefully straighten your front knee. Turn your trunk through ninety degrees so that you face forwards and your feet return to parallel. Repeat on the opposite side.

Caution: as you turn your body through ninety degrees (see Fig. 2) it is important to rotate your back foot through an angle of around sixty degrees. The reason for this is to avoid strain to the knee of your back leg as you turn your pelvis to face squarely forwards. If the angle through which you turn your back foot is too shallow, there will be a twisting effect on the back knee joint. Also, make sure that you turn your pelvis sufficiently to face squarely forwards over your front leg (see Fig. 2) before moving into the full posture. This is to avoid strain to your lower back due to twisting as you extend your arms and trunk.

The Standing Twist

The Standing Twist involves rotating the trunk from the stable base of legs and pelvis. The twisting action develops a flexible spine, improving upper body mobility as well as contributing to core strength.

1. Take a wide stride of approximately one metre with feet parallel and toes in line. Take your hands to your hips.
2. Turn your trunk to the right through an angle of ninety degrees so that your right foot faces forwards and your left foot rotates through an angle of around sixty degrees. Adjust your feet so that your

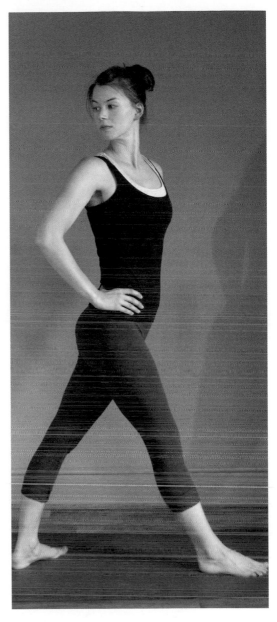

The Standing Twist Pose.

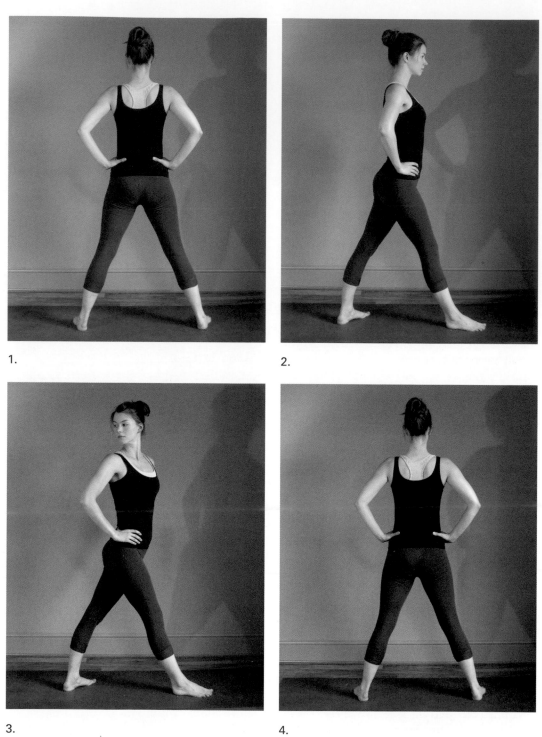

1.

2.

3.

4.

front heel is in line with your back ankle. Bring the left side of your pelvis round so that your pelvis faces squarely forwards over your front leg. Engage your thigh muscles and stabilize your pelvis keeping your tailbone long. Keep your sternum up, your abdomen long and flat and your head in central balance.

3. Inhale, then as you exhale, turn your trunk to the right and look over your right shoulder. Make sure that you do not rotate your pelvis – keep it facing squarely forwards with your feet firmly on the mat. Roll your shoulders down and back and keep your chest full, broad and active, abdomen long and flat. Breathe freely and hold the posture with full awareness and internal calm.

4. Release carefully turning your head, trunk, pelvis and feet and return to your starting position with feet parallel. Repeat on opposite side.

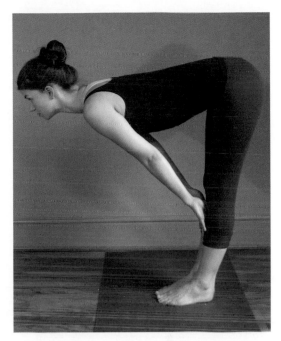

Gazing Posture.

Caution: whilst holding the posture keep your face and neck relaxed. As you release, take care not to jerk your head. Turn your head gently and with smooth motion so as not strain the neck vertebrae.

The Standing Forward Bend

A useful posture to complete your standing routine. It gives a strong stretch to the back of the body whilst releasing the trunk and relaxing the spine.

1. Commence in Mountain Pose.
2. Inhaling, raise your arms (this has the effect of extending the body opening the shoulder joints and releasing the spine). Take a couple of breaths.
3. Inhale keeping your sternum up. Exhaling, lead with the crown of your head and lower your trunk by pivoting from your pelvis. Take your fingers onto the front of your shins and look

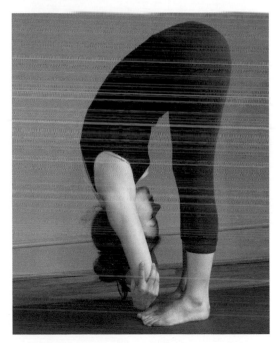

Full Posture.

forwards. This is known as 'Gazing Posture' which you should hold for two to three breaths. Keep your chest broad, your back long and flat (or slightly concave) and take care not to hyperextend the backs of your knees.

4. Inhale, then exhaling, move into the full posture allowing your trunk and head to release in front of your legs. Fold your arms below your head and allow your trunk to 'dangle'. Breathe freely taking several breaths and maintain full awareness and internal calm.

5. To release, reverse the movements. Inhaling and leading with the crown of

Standing Forward Bend.

1.

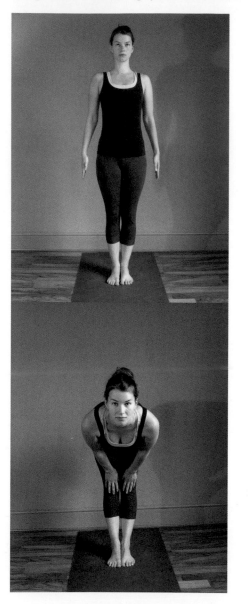

2.

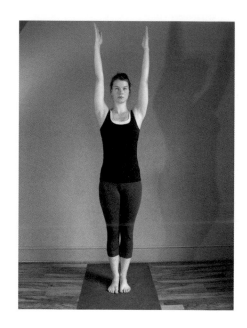

3.

your head, move into Gazing Posture before returning to Mountain pose.

Caution: as you bend forwards your pelvis will tilt backwards and upwards causing your hamstrings to stretch. Be mindful of your hamstrings. Overstretch can be avoided by softening (bending slightly) your knees particularly when moving into the posture and releasing from it. Also, avoid leaning back with your body weight in your heels (see Fig. 6) as this can cause strain to the hamstrings. Keep your weight forwards so that you are equally balanced on your heels and balls of feet (see Fig. 4).

4.

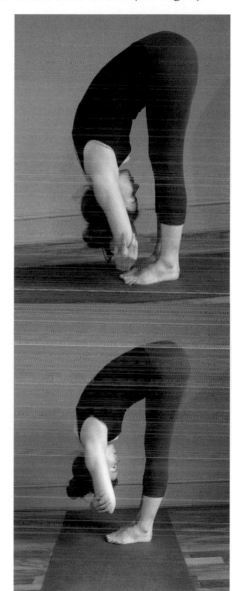

5.

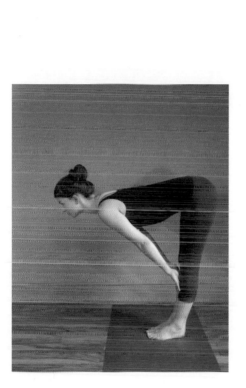

6. Incorrect.

65

5   The Seated Practice

The standing postures focus on body alignment and balance and deepen our awareness of anatomical structure. The seated postures function more at the physiological level, exercising our deeper muscles and refreshing our internal organs as well as improving the functioning of our bodily systems including digestive, circulatory, lymphatic, hormone and nervous systems. The seated postures are conducive to relaxation and although they may be practised at any time, are especially beneficial in the evening when we need to wind down after the day's activities.

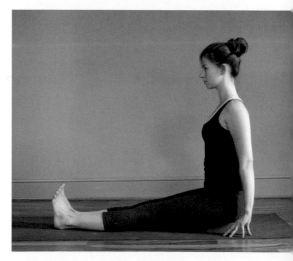

The Staff Pose. 1.

The Staff Pose
A seated posture symbolizing the firmness and support of a staff or stick.

1. Sit on the mat or on a single block with your legs extended. Keep your feet together with your soles squarely forwards. Spread your toes and push the balls of your feet slightly away, keeping your inner ankles soft. Engage your thigh muscles allowing the backs of your knees to gently open but take care not to hyperextend. Come onto the front of your sitting bones and take a few moments to establish your foundation.
2. Place your hands by the sides of your hips and prepare to align your trunk. Inhaling, lift your sternum and roll your shoulders down and back so that your chest is full,

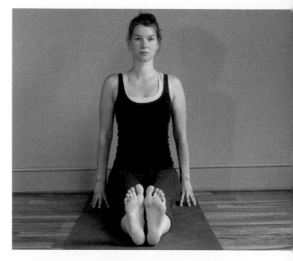

2.

broad and active, your abdomen long and flat. Feel the release of your spine as your back lengthens. Bring your head into central balance and look straight ahead, eyes open and focus soft and breathe freely, holding the posture with full awareness.

Modification: if you feel the need for support, sit with your back against a wall. Ensure that your pelvis is flush with the skirting board and that your trunk and the back of your head make contact with the wall.

The Upward Cobbler and Resting Cobbler Poses

The Upward Cobbler resembles the position adopted by the ancient, Indian cobbler. The posture develops a strong back with release of the spine and also improves flexibility in the pelvic joints. The Resting Cobbler is a forward bend that improves flexibility in the back and spine and brings suppleness to the pelvic joints.

1. Commence in Staff Pose sitting on the mat or on one block.
2. Bend your knees and taking hold of your ankles, bring your heels in close to your pelvis allowing your knees to roll out to the sides. Place the soles of your feet together and clasp your toes, with your little fingers under your little toes. Moving onto the front of your sitting bones take a few moments to establish your base. Inhaling, lift your sternum and roll your shoulders down and back so that your chest is full, broad and active, your abdomen long and flat. Feel the release of your spine as your back lengthens. Bring your head into central balance and look straight ahead with eyes open, focus soft and hold the posture with full awareness for several breaths.
3. Prepare to move into the Resting Cobbler Pose. Place your thumbs on the insides of the soles of your feet, fingers on the outsides. Bend your elbows out to the sides so that they rest on your inner thighs. Turn the soles of your feet outwards and

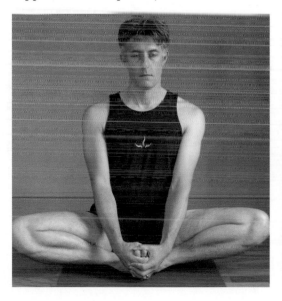

The Upward Cobbler Pose.

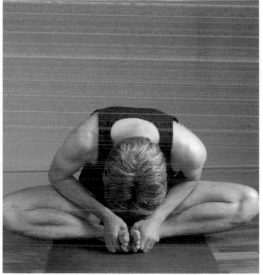

The Resting Cobbler Pose.

upwards (as if you are opening the pages of a book) and pressing your elbows gently against your inner thighs, ease your trunk forwards and release your head. Hold the posture for three to four breaths, maintaining inner calm.

To release, inhale as you lift your head, chest and trunk, returning to Upward Cobbler Pose. Release your hands and straighten your legs, returning to Staff Pose.

Modification: sit with your back against a wall for additional support. Make sure that your pelvis is flush with the skirting board and that the back of your body is fully supported by the wall.

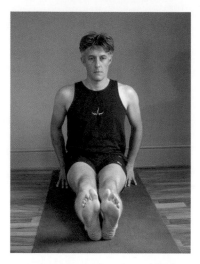

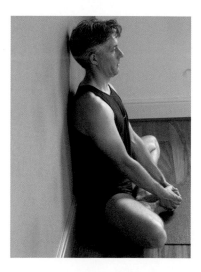

The Upward and Resting Cobbler Poses. 1.

2.

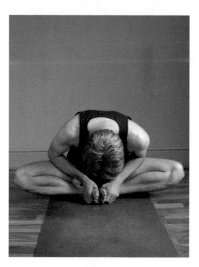

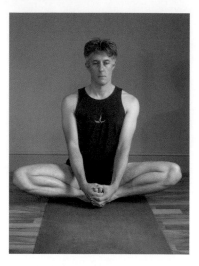

3.

Modification.

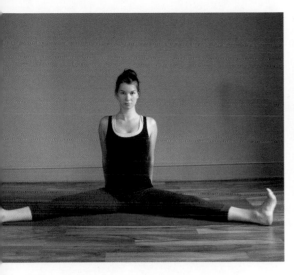

The Wide Angle Pose: upward stage.

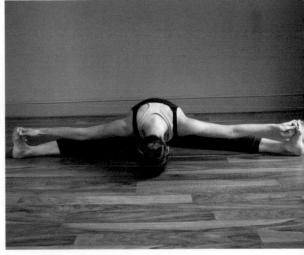

The Wide Angle Pose: forward bend.

The Wide Angle Pose

This has two stages: an upward stage that develops a strong back and spinal release as well as flexibility in the pelvic joints; and a second stage – a forward bend that improves flexibility in the back, spine and pelvic joints. The inner thigh muscles also receive a good stretch. The posture benefits from a broad, stable base.

1. Commence in Staff Pose.
2. Take your feet into a wide stride. Keep your heels to the same horizontal plane and turn your toes up to the ceiling so that you are resting on your calf muscles. Engage your thigh muscles allowing the backs of your knees to gently open (taking care not to hyperextend). Come onto the front of your sitting bones and take a few moments to establish your base. Rest your hands on your hips.
3. Take your hands behind you and with fingers pointing forwards, push your fingers under your buttocks or upper thighs. Lift your sternum and roll your shoulders down and back so that your chest is full, broad and active, your abdomen long and flat and feel the release of your spine as your back lengthens. Bring your head into central balance and look straight ahead with eyes open, focus soft and breathe freely holding the posture with full awareness and inner calm.
4. To move into the forward bend, 'walk' your hands along the floor in front of you and leading with your chest, bring your trunk forwards and release your head.
5. Take your arms out to the sides and clasp either your shins or, if you can reach, your big toes, taking hold of them with index and middle fingers.
6. To release, inhale as you lift your head, chest and trunk returning to upright. Bring your heels together as you return to Staff Pose.

Caution: in both Cobbler and Wide Angle Poses, avoid overstretching. This is particularly important during the forward bends. If you are not very flexible you will find that you cannot bend very far. This is fine: be

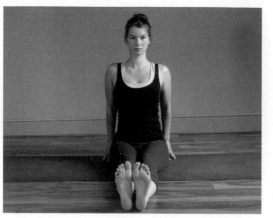

The Wide Angle Pose.

1.

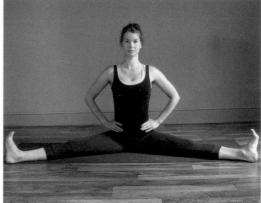

2.

3.

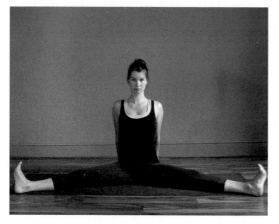

patient. Your flexibility will improve with time and practice, so do not rush the process. In all postures it is important that you do not push yourself beyond your limit. Bear in mind that it is the quality rather than the quantity of your stretch that is important.

The next group of postures are often performed in sequence, and comprise seated forward bends, backbends and twists.

By doing these postures in succession, we bring balance and harmony to the body, bending in different and complementary ways. The postures are simultaneously energizing and relaxing.

Know your limit

As the term 'Forward Bend' implies, we are bending the trunk of the body forwards over the pelvis and legs. The

4.

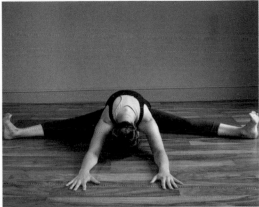

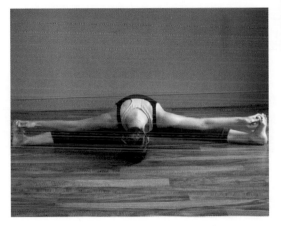

5.

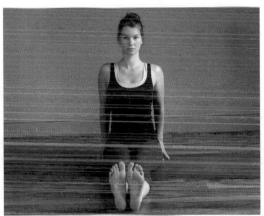

6.

effect is to extend the back of the body whilst 'closing' the front. As we become more flexible our ability to bend improves. The process is subtle and requires patience. We must resist the urge to push ahead too quickly and risk strain or injury. This applies to all postures. With practice we are able to feel when we have reached our limit or maximum stretch. This 'limit' will shift as our flexibility improves. It is at this moment of finding our limit that we play the edge. In other words, we bring challenge to our posture by making subtle adjustments to promote activity, whilst at the same time exercise appropriate caution to avoid overstretch and risk of injury. The process of knowing how to finely tune our posture to obtain maximum benefit develops with experience.

Forward bends

The Head to Knee Pose

This provides a strong stretch to the back of the body bringing flexibility to the back and release of the spine. The trunk is extended over the legs and pelvis.

1. Commence in Staff Pose, sitting on one block.
2. Bend your right leg, taking your knee out to the side and clasping your ankle, bring your right heel in close to your groin and rest the ball of your right foot against or slightly under your inner, left thigh. Take your knee down to rest on the mat (see 'Caution' below). Come onto the front of your sitting bones and align your trunk to face your straight left leg.
3. Take a folded belt and holding it in both hands, place it around the sole of your left foot. Pull on the belt and leading with your chest, lean your trunk slightly forwards pivoting from your pelvis. Inhaling, lift your sternum and keeping your chest up push your spine into your back so that your back is long and erect. Look up to the ceiling and relax your face and forehead. Hold the stretch with full awareness for two to three breaths.

The Head to Knee Pose.

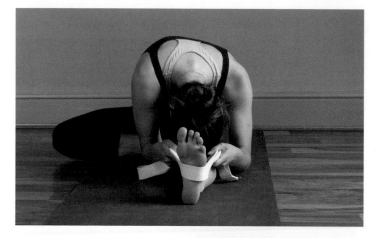

1.

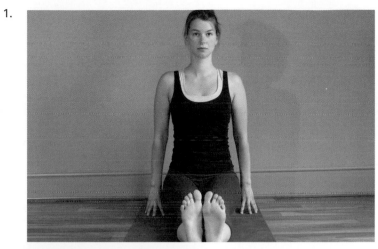

2.

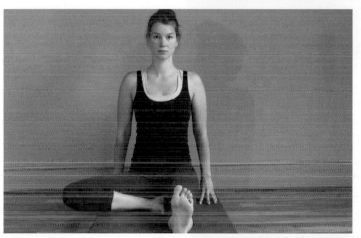

3.

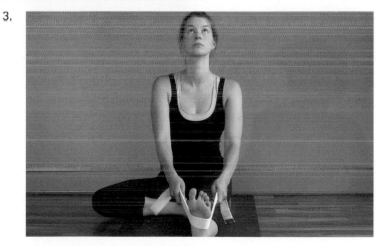

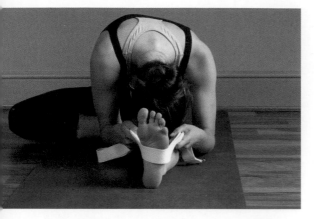

4.

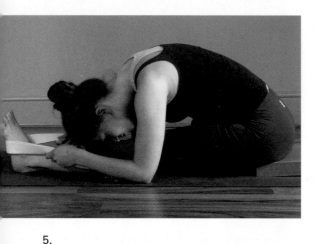

5.

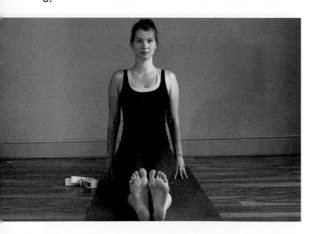

6.

4. Inhale. Then, exhaling, bring your trunk forwards over your straight leg. Lead with your chest and work your hands up the belt towards your foot as you move into the bend. It may take three to four breaths to bring you into your optimum stretch, as you settle further into the posture with each exhalation. Release your head to face your knee.
5. Breathe freely and hold with full awareness, maintaining inner calm.
6. To release, reverse the movements. Inhaling, lift your head, chest and trunk and slide your hands back up the belt as you return to upright. Release your belt and return to Staff Pose. Repeat on other side.

Caution: if your bent knee does not rest comfortably down on the mat it is important to support it, to protect the knee joint from strain or injury. This can be done with blocks or books etc. Ensure that the support is placed under the actual knee joint – not under the shin.

As you extend your trunk over your straight leg there will be a slight backwards tilt of your pelvis causing the hamstrings of your straight leg to stretch. If you feel strain in the hamstrings, slightly soften the knee. If the strain persists you may need to reduce the extent of your forward bend. Avoid overstretching.

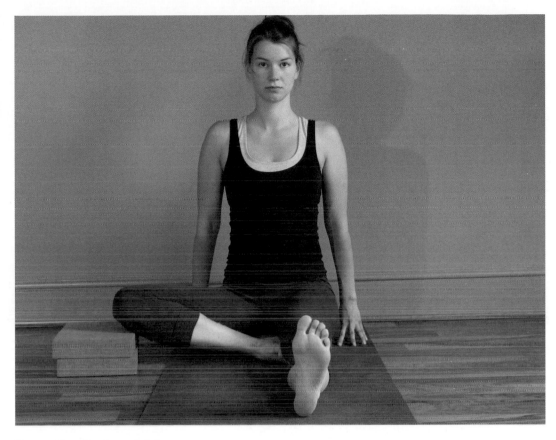

Supporting the knee joint.

The Seated Forward Bend (pages 76–7)

This bend has similar benefits to the Head to Knee Pose although it provides a stronger stretch.

1. Commence in Staff Pose sitting on one block. Keep your feet together with soles squarely forwards and engage your thigh muscles, gently opening the backs of your knees but taking care not to hyperextend. Come onto the front of your sitting bones.
2. Place a folded belt round the soles of your feet and hold in both hands. Pull on the belt and leading with your chest, bring your trunk slightly forwards pivoting from your pelvis. Inhaling, lift your sternum and keeping your chest up push your spine into your back so that your back is long and erect.
3. Look up to the ceiling and keep your face and forehead relaxed. Hold for two to three breaths with full awareness and inner calm.
4. Inhale. Then, exhaling, bring your trunk forwards over your legs and pelvis. As you extend, lead with your chest and work your hands up the belt towards your feet. It may take three to four breaths before you reach your optimum stretch as you settle further into the posture with each exhalation.

Release your head to face your legs.
5. Breathe freely and hold with full awareness, maintaining inner calm.
6. To release, reverse the movements. Inhale

as you lift your head, chest and trunk and
slide your hands back up the belt as you
return to upright. Release the belt
returning to Staff Pose.

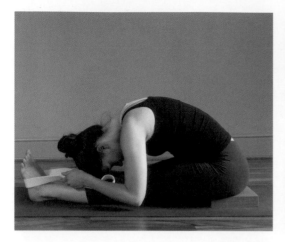

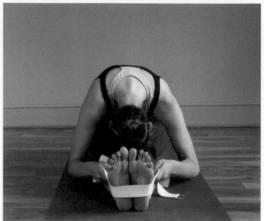

The Seated Forward Bend.

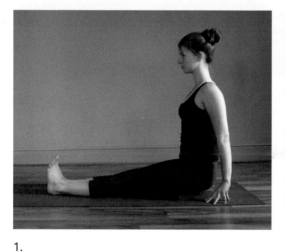

1.

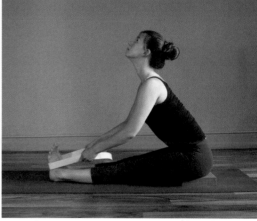

2.

Caution: as you bring your trunk forwards there will be a slight backwards tilt of your pelvis causing your hamstrings to stretch. If you feel strain in the hamstrings, slightly 'soften' your knees to avoid overstretch. If you still feel strain you may need to reduce the extent of your forward bend. Avoid over-stretching.

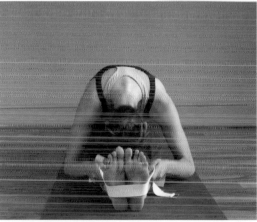

3.

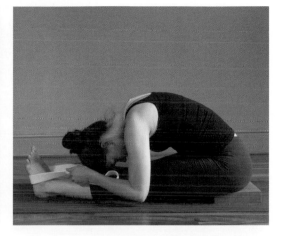

4.

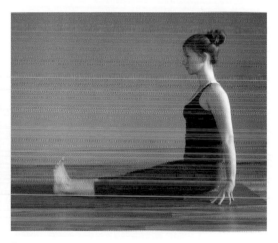

5.

6.

6   Backbends and Twists

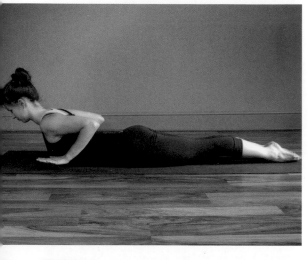

Half Cobra.

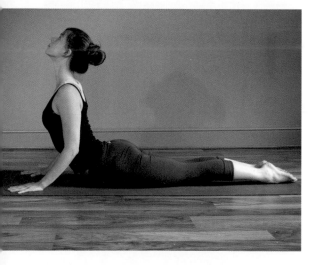

Full Cobra.

The forward bends provide a stretch to the back of the body while the front of the body 'closes'. To restore physical balance, it is necessary to reverse the movement. The backbends complement the forward bends by lengthening and broadening the front of the body whilst the back is gently arched so that the spine assumes an inwards curve. It is this counter-movement that restores body balance. The backbends are rejuvenating postures which are particularly good for strengthening the back and developing a flexible spine as well as toning the abdomen.

The Cobra Pose
This pose resembles the poisonous, hooded snake of India.

1. Lie on the front of your body face down. Take your legs slightly apart and rest on the tops of your feet. Engage your thigh muscles allowing the backs of your knees to gently open and your knee caps to lift off the mat. Place your hands palms down by the sides of your rib cage, your elbows tucked in to your sides. The upper and lower arms should form right angles at the inner elbow joints.
2. Inhaling, slide your nose forwards along the mat and lift your head and top chest whilst keeping your lower rib crest down on the mat for support. Roll your shoulders down and back and keep your top chest full and broad with your shoulder

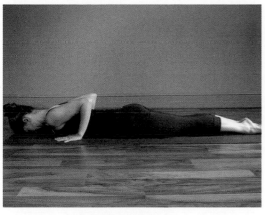

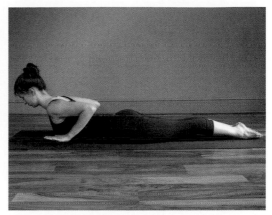

The Cobra Pose. 1.

2.

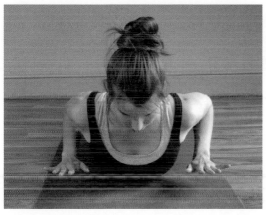

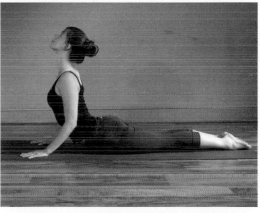

3.

4.

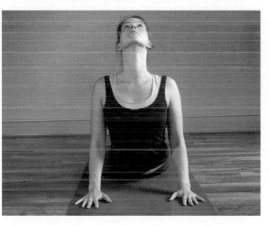

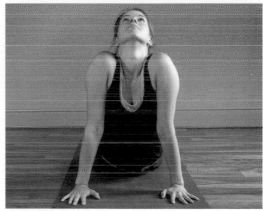

5.

6. Incorrect.

blades pressing into your back. Lift your palms off the mat and take two to three breaths holding the posture with awareness and inner calm. This is the Half Cobra.

3. During the holding stage keep your legs strong with thigh muscles engaged. Feel the lengthening of your abdomen and the gentle arching of your spine in your back. Do not strain. To release, exhale as you return to face down position.

4. To move into Full Cobra, come up firstly into Half Cobra. Inhale, then exhaling, push on the palms of your hands and allow your elbow joints to open as you lift your chest and lengthen your abdomen whilst keeping the front of your pelvis firmly on the mat. As you move into the Full Cobra, gently coax your spine to arch further into your back.

5. Roll your shoulders down and back and keep your chest full, broad and

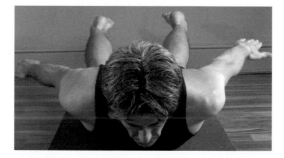

The Locust Pose.

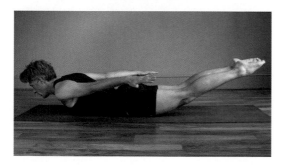

active, your abdomen long and flat. Direct your gaze upwards and breathe freely as you hold the pose with awareness and inner calm. When you are ready to release, exhale and slowly return to face down position.

Caution: it is important to keep your legs strong with your thigh muscles engaged throughout the posture. This is to prevent undue strain in the lower back. Also, keep your tail bone long and do not harden your back muscles. Do not lift your shoulders (see Fig. 6) – keep your neck long and free. Do not attempt the Full Cobra until you are fully confident in the Half Cobra. The Full Cobra is a strong posture which requires a flexible spine, so take the process slowly and carefully, adjusting your stretch in accordance with your flexibility. This is to avoid the risk of strain or injury to your lower back. It may take time and practice before you are flexible enough for the full stage.

The Locust Pose

This has the appearance of the winged insect that migrates in swarms and is native to Africa and Asia. Like the Cobra, the Locust Pose is a backbend, which develops a strong back and a flexible spine.

1. Lie on your mat face down. Extend your arms, placing them underneath you with fists clenched and knuckles of thumbs in contact. With your arms underneath you your clenched fingers and thumbs should press against your pubic bone. Roll from side to side moving your elbows under your trunk. Take your legs slightly apart and rest on the tops of your feet. Engage your thigh muscles allowing the backs of your knees to gently open and your knee caps to lift off the mat.

2. Raise your right leg just a few inches off the mat, keeping your leg strong and

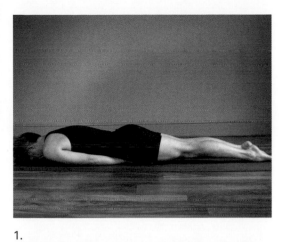

1.

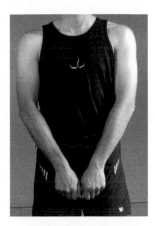

Hands position.

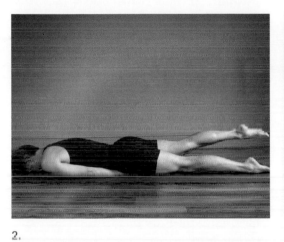

2.

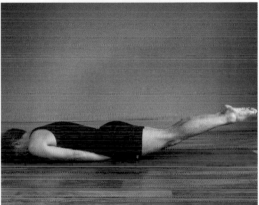

3. Half locust.

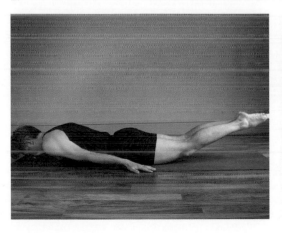

4.

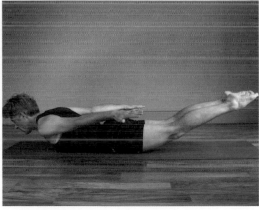

5. Full locust.

extending into your toes. Hold for two to three breaths before releasing. Repeat with the opposite leg.

3. Raise both legs keeping them strong and straight and extend into your toes. Keep your head down on the mat. This is the Half Locust Pose. Hold with full awareness and internal calm for two to three breaths before releasing. Repeat.

4. Release your arms and extend them by your sides, palms facing down.

5. Inhaling, raise your head, hands arms and top chest and pull back with your arms so that your top chest is full and broad and your shoulder blades press into your back. Exhaling, raise both legs keeping them strong and straight as you extend into your toes. Encourage your spine to arch gently into your back taking care not to harden your back muscles. This is the Full Locust Pose. Hold with full awareness and internal calm for three to four breaths, before releasing and returning to face down position. Repeat the pose.

Caution: do not harden your back muscles. By keeping your thigh muscles engaged throughout the posture, you help prevent strain to the lower back. Come out of the pose if you feel strain.

Backbends require a flexible spine and as with all postures, it is wise to proceed carefully and patiently so as to avoid strain. After back bending it is good practice to rest your back and spine before moving on to your next posture.

The Child Pose

An excellent posture for resting the lower back, which is particularly susceptible to strain. The pose resembles the position adopted by small children when they are feeling tired.

1. From lying face down push up onto your hands and knees. Put your big toes together and separate your heels (as in Down Hero Pose described earlier). Push your pelvis backwards and downwards until it rests on your heels. Release your head and rest your forehead on the mat. Bring your arms round by your shins, palms facing upwards and allow your back to open and round. Breathe freely and keeping your face and forehead relaxed, hold the posture with full awareness, allowing your back to settle and rest.

Caution: if your pelvis does not rest comfortably on your heels you risk placing strain in the knee joints. If this is the case, place a block(s) or folded blanket on your heels to support your pelvis. Also, avoid strain to the head and neck and if necessary support your forehead on a block or blocks (see Modification 1). If you feel uncomfortable in the head-down position, then reverse the posture. Lie on your back whilst gently squeezing your knees in towards your chest and relax (see Modification 2). This has a similar recuperating effect to the Child Pose.

The Inclined Plane Pose

The Inclined Plane is also complementary to the forward bends. It strengthens the front of the torso and the wrists as well as strengthening the back and bringing flexibility to the spine.

1. Commence in Staff Pose. Lean back taking your weight onto your hands. Keep your thigh muscles engaged and your head in central balance with your chin tucked in slightly. Lift your sternum and roll your shoulders down and back so that your chest is full, broad and active, your abdomen long, firm and flat. Feel your shoulder blades pressing into your upper back. Encourage your spine to arch gently

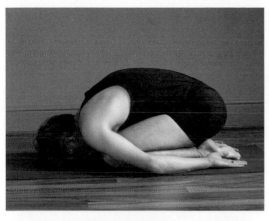

The Child Pose. 1.

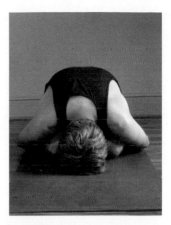

Allow back to open and round.

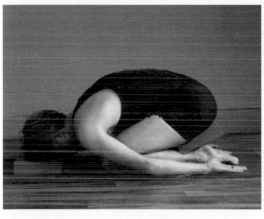

Modification 1.

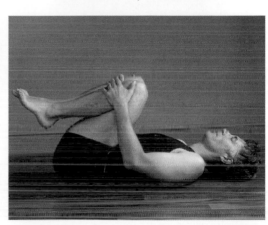

Modification 2.

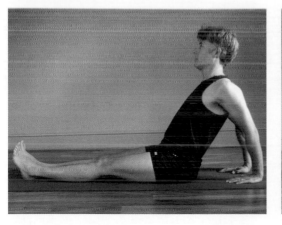

Gentle backbend: stage 1.

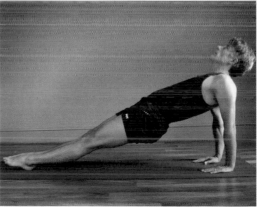

Full Inclined Plane.

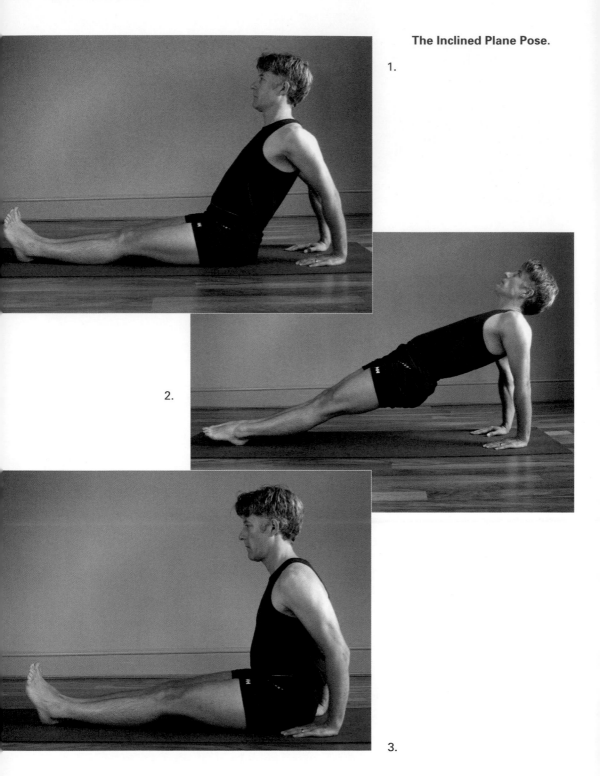

The Inclined Plane Pose.

1.

2.

3.

into your back and hold the posture for three to four breaths with full awareness and internal calm.

2. Push on your palms and lift your pelvis, turning the soles of your feet towards the mat. Direct your gaze to the ceiling. Keep your face relaxed, your chest broad, abdomen long, firm and flat and your tail bone long. Hold with full awareness and internal calm for three to four breaths before releasing.

3. Return to Staff Pose.

   To recuperate, lie on your back with your knees pulled in towards your chest (see Modification 2 above). Keep your face relaxed and breathe freely, allowing your back to fully settle before moving on.

Caution: the full posture requires a strong back and flexible wrists. Take care to avoid strain in your back and in your wrists.

Ensure that you are proficient in the first stage before moving on to the Full Inclined Plane Pose.

The Twists

The twists are a group of postures which involve rotating the spine; regular practice brings spinal flexibility and increased mobility to the trunk. They help tone the spinal and abdominal muscles as well as improving spinal blood flow and refreshing the spinal nerves. The twists can be practised from seated, standing, lying or inverted positions. They are often performed in combination with forward bends and backbends, completing the sequence.

The Torso Stretch

A gentle, seated twist which — as the name suggests — stretches and tones the torso.

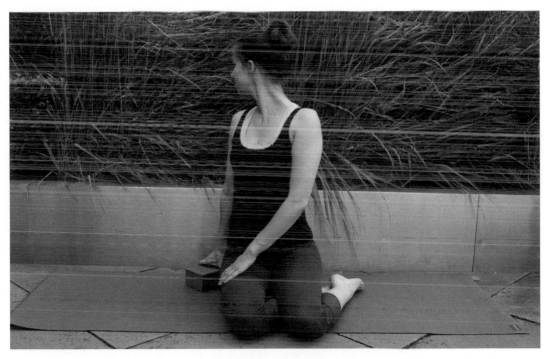

The Torso Stretch.

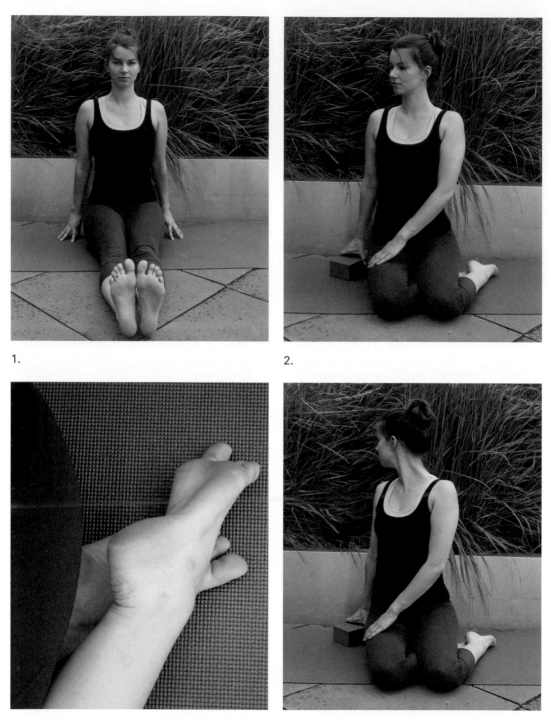

1.

2.

Position of feet.

3.

1. Commence in Staff Pose sitting on a block. Place a further block or similar support obliquely, behind your right hip.

2. Swing your feet round to the left and bring your knees together in front of you so that they rest on the mat. The top of your left foot should rest on the sole of your right foot. Take hold of your ankles and gently pull your feet a little further round to the left. Place your right hand on the block behind your right hip – this is to provide support as you lengthen your trunk and allow the release of your spine. Place your left hand on your right thigh. Keep your chest up, shoulders rolling down and back so that your chest is full, broad and active, your abdomen long and flat. Keep your back erect, head in central balance and direct your gaze forwards.

3. Inhaling, lift your sternum and then exhale as you turn your trunk to the right. Inhale again and exhaling, roll your shoulders back and turn your head gently to look over your right shoulder. Breathe freely and hold the posture for three to four breaths, with awareness and internal calm. To release, gently turn your head and your trunk to face forwards before releasing your legs to return to Staff Pose.

Now, reposition your block (or similar support) to lie obliquely behind your left hip and repeat the pose on other side, this time swinging your feet round to the right.

Caution: it is important that your trunk is erect and your spine fully released before turning your body and moving into the twist. Supporting yourself with hands or fingertips on the support behind your hip enables you to lengthen your trunk so that your spine is fully released. Always be careful when turning your head whilst moving into and coming out of the posture. Never jerk your head, always keep the movement smooth. Women should avoid seated twists during menstruation.

Note: The blocks, belts, blankets we use are referred to as props. The wall, when it is used to aid balance and alignment is also a 'prop'. The intention of using props is to provide support whilst we are developing our skills in posture work. As you become more adept in your yoga practice your confidence will build, as will your strength and flexibility, and you might find you no longer need to use the props. Use the aids sensibly and if they cease to be of help to your practice you may decide to stop using them

7   The Final Relaxation

When you have completed the active part of your yoga practice it is wise to rest for a short time so that you can enjoy and appreciate the sensations of well-being that have developed as a result of your practice. It is a time to cool down and settle your mind before continuing with life's routine.

The secret of good relaxation is in the ability to 'let go'. In the West there is the tendency to be always doing and to be on the go. The idea of 'non doing' can be a difficult concept in our Western culture where being busy and continually active equate with importance and high status. Yet this is to deny the joy of freedom. Taking the opportunity to simply do nothing and to let go is not about being lazy or shirking responsibilities. It is about embracing the moment, giving free rein to our thoughts, feelings and emotions without distractions and without pressures. A few minutes of proper relaxation will restore harmony so that we are more efficient and useful as we continue our daily activities.

To wind down after your yoga session, sit in Easy Pose or Adepts Pose or lie on your back in Corpse Pose for two to three minutes or longer. Exercise tends to raise the body temperature and this may fall quite quickly as you relax. You may wish to put on your socks or a jumper or, if you are lying down, perhaps cover yourself with a blanket.

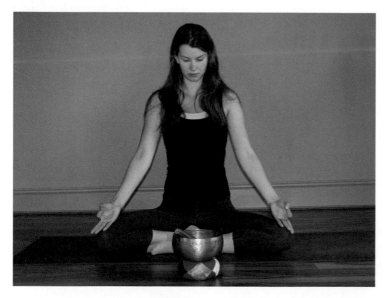

Resting in Adept's Pose.

After a long session you will probably prefer to relax for five to ten minutes on your back in Corpse Pose. Follow the procedure described earlier and allow yourself to fully settle on your mat. A useful technique for letting go is to bring conscious awareness to the sensations in your body and to your breath. And to bring together the contrasting states of stability and feeling secure on the one hand, lightness and freedom on the other.

Relaxing in Corpse Pose

1. Bring awareness to the contact that the back of your body is making with the mat to include the back of your head, shoulder blades, trunk, pelvis, legs, calves and heels. Feel the support underneath your shoulders, arms and hands. Surrender to the gravitational pull on your body as if you are sinking into the ground. Let go. Allow yourself to experience the sensations of being supported, grounded, down to earth. Stay with and embrace these sensations for several breaths.

2. Shift attention to your body surface. Allow the muscles of your face to soften relaxing your eyes, eyelids, bridge of nose, cheeks, lips and tongue root. If you are clenching your teeth allow your lower jaw to relax so that your teeth slightly separate. Soften your throat. Focus on your chest and envisage your heart opening

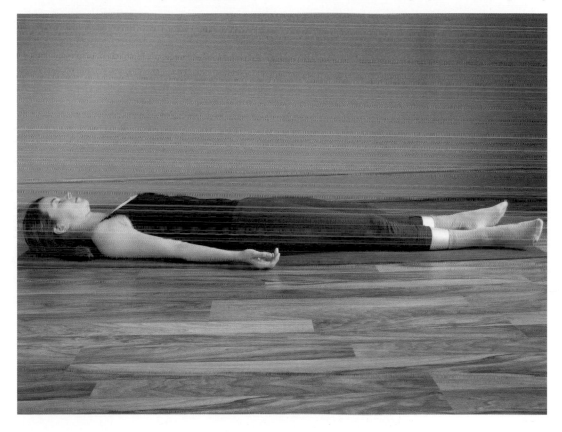

The Corpse Pose.

and your chest expanding so that you experience the sensations of lightness and being free. Let the feeling of lightness infiltrate your abdomen and pelvis. Notice if you are tensing the muscles in your pelvis floor and if so, let go. Allow your palms to soften and observe how your fingers lightly curl as you relax. Stay with and embrace these sensations.

3. Spend a few minutes in silence in full awareness of your breath and of the subtle sensations and changes in your body as you let go and allow yourself to be completely at ease.

The Final Release

Do not come out of your relaxation suddenly. Take your time, releasing carefully and attentively. If you are in Corpse Pose, gently roll your head from side to side for several repetitions. Now bend your knees and squeeze them in towards your chest. Roll on your back, clockwise, anticlockwise, side to side and back and forth. Enjoy the massaging effect on your back and spine. Finally roll onto your right side, taking your right arm behind you and raising your knee. Stay on your side for a few moments until you are ready to come up then ease yourself to sitting.

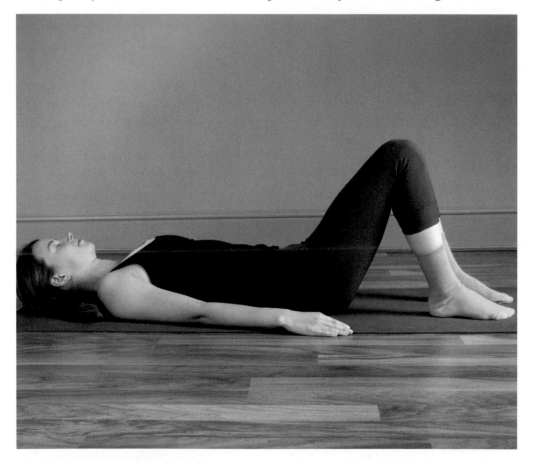

Release slowly.

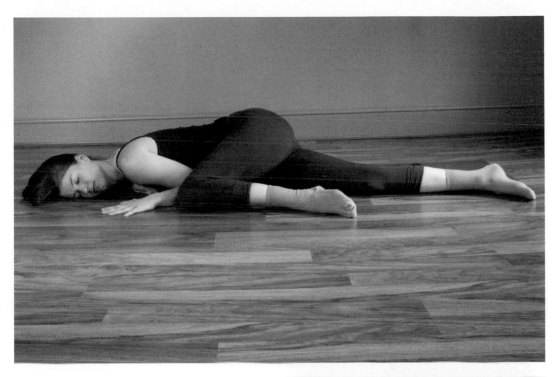

ABOVE: Recovery.

RIGHT: Om Shanti ('peace be with you').

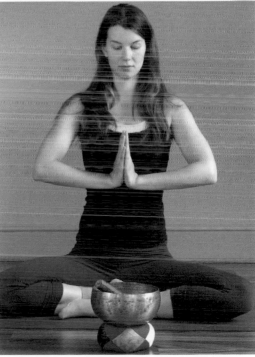

8   The Breath

Breath is life. The very first action of an infant at birth is to take a breath in – to inspire. This inspiration represents the first moment of life outside the womb. The final action of a living being is to breathe out – to expire. This expiration signifies the end of life as we know it. From the moment of birth until the instant of death we breathe. It is our breath that keeps us alive. Our breath is constant and as well as sustaining life, it becomes a useful object on which we can focus our attention with the aim of bringing steadiness of mind. Working with the breath is very much a part of yoga practice.

Why do we breathe?

Firstly, there is the physiological requirement of breathing to keep us alive. We need oxygen from the air to nourish all our bodily cells, tissues and organs so that our body can perform its many functions properly and efficiently. The oxygen in the air we breathe is transferred from our lungs to our arterial bloodstream where it is carried to every cell in our body. This oxygen is vital to cell function. Conversely, the waste product of cellular metabolism, carbon dioxide, needs to be eliminated from our body. The carbon dioxide is transported in our venous blood to be transferred to the lungs and is removed from our body each time we breathe out. Yoga postures develop the parts of our body that are concerned with the mechanism of breathing, including the muscles of the chest and abdomen. Yoga helps to improve our lung capacity and in association with our ability to withstand stress, leads to more efficient breathing.

Next, our emotions are linked to our breath. When we get excited or become angry and upset, our breathing tends to become rapid and shallow. By making the conscious effort to slow down and deepen our breath, we become calmer. Most of us have experienced this when taking a few deep breaths prior to moving into a stressful situation such as a job interview, or sitting an important examination, not to mention giving birth. It is our breathing that helps to calm us down. Sometimes, after a sudden shock or fright, our breath is temporarily suspended. There is a connection between our breathing and our nervous system and in yoga, we are taught to focus on our breath and to regulate it with the purpose of bringing steadiness of mind.

And lastly, there is the issue of prana, which can be interpreted as energy, life force, vitality. It is a yogic concept that is sometimes difficult for the average Westerner to grasp. This is because, like many yogic beliefs, the presence of prana is not qualified by scientific evidence. The yogic idea is that in addition to the physical body as we know it in its anatomical and physiological forms, we also have a 'subtle' body and it is in this 'layer' that life force in the form of pranic energy exists and circulates. Prana is said to exist everywhere: in the air we breathe, in the water we drink, in the food we eat. It is said to be transported in the subtle body in thousands of channels called nadis of which there are three main channels: Ida, Pingala, and Sushuma associated with the spinal cord. It is believed that the yoga postures help conserve our pranic energy and keep it circulating. The nadis (channels) can become blocked due to poor health, lack of fitness, stress and anything that is an obstacle to our overall well being. The practice of yoga helps keep the nadis open so that prana can flow freely. As long as our energy is not squandered and the nadis remain open, then prana flows freely and abundantly in our body and we feel energized.

Yoga and breath

To breathe well and efficiently we need to be relaxed. Our ability to relax is enhanced if our body is fit and healthy, our mind steady and calm. These qualities are acquired through yoga. The subject of breath 'regulation' is referred to as pranayama. Pranayama is profound and diverse – an in-depth study is outside the scope of this book. Nevertheless, it is essential that we understand the fundamental principles of how to breathe in our yoga practice and these will be discussed.

As a general rule, movements that involve extending or 'opening' the front of the body correspond with taking a breath in – inhalation. Conversely, movements involved with 'closing' the front of the body, with breathing out – exhalation. Here are some examples:

Raising the arms (see Fig. 1) establishes

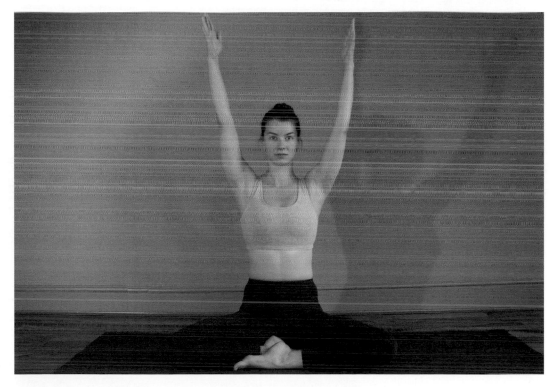

1. Inhale (arms raised).

'opening' and extending the front of the body and therefore corresponds with a breath in. Conversely lowering the arms (see Fig. 2) involves breathing out. In the seated Forward Bend (see Fig. 3), moving into the posture involves 'closing' the front of the body and is synchronized with breathing out; releasing from the posture (see Fig. 4) is an 'opening' movement involving a breath in.

The illustrations apply to opening and closing movements associated with going into and coming out of postures. We also need to know how to breathe when holding postures. During the holding stage we breathe freely and fully giving full attention to the sensations in our body. With each inhalation we bring 'vitality' to our body and with each exhalation a letting go or 'release' as we ease further into our posture. It is with this regular process of action and release to coincide with inhaling and exhaling, that we are able to contain our pranic energy and keep it flowing so that we remain simultaneously energized and relaxed. As we become more familiar and at ease with yoga our breathing will improve and we will come to experience the subtlety of the process.

2. Exhale (arms lowered).

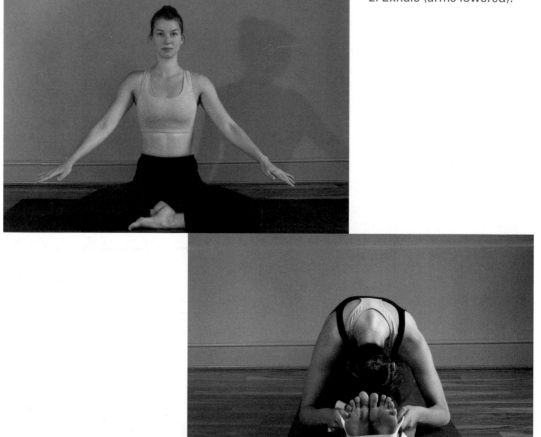

3. Exhale (bending forwards).

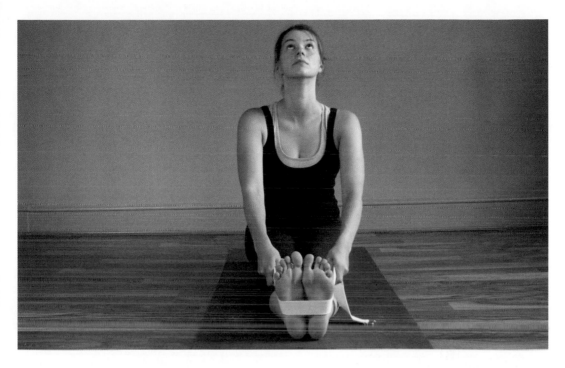

ABOVE: 4. Inhale (raising trunk).

BELOW: Relaxed action.

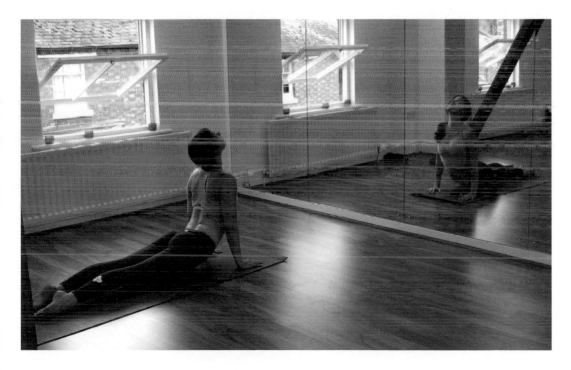

The mechanics of breathing

During normal, quiet breathing when we are relaxed we tend to breathe mainly with the diaphragm. This is a dome shaped muscle that occupies the floor of the chest cavity, separating the thorax from the abdomen. As we inhale, the muscular dome descends and flattens exerting pressure in the abdominal cavity; this causes the abdominal wall to expand, a bit like the expansion when we inflate a balloon. At the same time, the flattening of the diaphragm creates an increase in volume in the chest cavity and the resulting differential pressure gradient between the air in the atmosphere and that in our lungs causes air to be drawn into the lungs. As we exhale, the abdominal wall moves inwards as the diaphragm returns to its dome shape, pushing up into the chest cavity. The simultaneous reduction in chest volume increases the pressure in the chest cavity causing air to be expelled from the lungs.

Caution: in all breathing exercises it is essential to avoid strain. Being relaxed is the secret of good breathing. Stop your practice if you feel dizzy, light headed or uncomfortable. It is important that you are proficient in your yoga postures before moving on to the breathing exercises.

Exercise: abdominal breathing

1. Sit comfortably on your mat in Easy Pose or Adepts Pose. Release your shoulders and relax your eyes, tongue root, lower jaw and pelvic floor. Gently, lift your sternum and bring your head into central balance. Place your palms on either sides of your abdomen.

2. When you are settled, inhale slowly through your nostrils and envisage that you are breathing into your abdomen. Do not move your chest. As your abdominal wall expands, feel your hands move outwards and further apart. As you let go and exhale, your hands will return to their former position as your abdominal wall flattens and releases. Repeat several times until you get the hang of it.

Note: Unless you are relaxed you may find that your chest is moving up and down or your abdominal wall moves in when it should be moving out and vice versa. With practice and the ability to relax, the exercise becomes easier.

As our activity increases, so does our body's need for oxygen. Also, the increased cellular activity during exercise produces more carbon dioxide which needs to be eliminated from our lungs. During moderate exercise, we automatically step up our breathing by utilizing the mid chest as well as the abdomen. This involves extending our inhalations from abdomen into mid chest. As this happens, our chest expands as our rib cage lifts upwards and outwards and this increases the volume of the chest cavity, allowing more air to enter our lungs. As we exhale, the chest, abdomen and diaphragm return to their former positions and the volume in the chest cavity is reduced as air is eliminated from our lungs.

Note: inhalation is an active process which requires muscular effort to increase the size of the abdominal and chest cavities, whereas exhalation is passive, involving a release and letting go.

Abdominal breathing exercise.

1.

2.

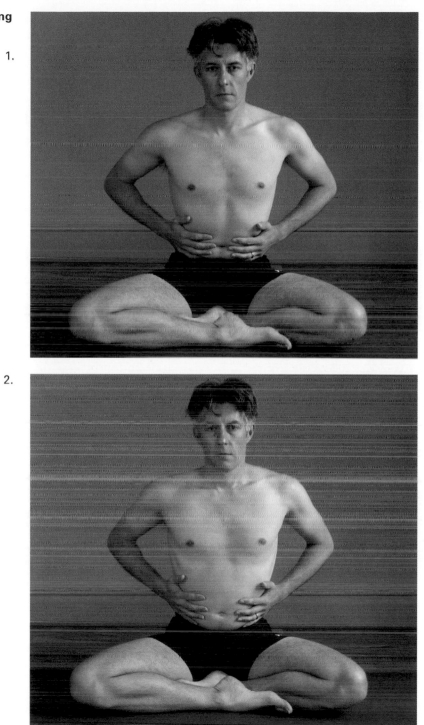

Exercise: mid chest breathing

1. Place your hands on either sides of your rib cage. Breathing through your nose, take a slightly longer and deeper inhalation than before. As you inhale, direct your breath initially to your abdomen then gently and without strain, extend your breath into your mid chest (rib cage). Your abdominal wall will expand initially, followed by the upward and outward movement of your rib cage.
2. The expansion of your mid chest will cause your hands to move outwards and further apart. As you exhale, your hands will return to their former position with the release of your rib cage.

As our activity increases still further – for example, if we are running, or doing a strenuous work-out in the gym, or partaking in one of the more aerobic styles of yoga – we need to utilize the full capacity of our lungs. This will involve not only abdominal and mid chest breathing, but also 'top chest'. Top chest breathing involves the lifting of the entire rib cage which is brought about by muscles which lift our clavicles (collar bones).

Exercise: top chest breathing

1. Place your fingers on your collar bones. Take a long deep inhalation through your nostrils directing your breath initially to your abdomen, extending to your mid chest and finally to your top chest.
2. As you reach the extent of your inhalation you will feel your collar bones lift as your entire rib cage is raised, allowing your lungs to fill to their full capacity. As you exhale, top chest, mid chest, and abdomen return spontaneously to their former position.

The Full Yoga Breath

When you have mastered the above exercises you will be ready for the Full Yoga Breath. This involves a slow, progressive transition from abdominal, to mid chest, to top chest breathing, enabling you to utilize your lungs to full capacity and in doing so, nourish your whole body. The exercise can be carried out from a comfortable seated posture but initially, it is better to practise lying on your back in Corpse Pose. Deepak Chopra and David Simon[5] refer to the process of consciously directing the breath to fill three different areas of the lungs, namely the lower, middle and upper regions to coincide with abdominal, mid chest and top chest breathing. The exercise is at the same time energizing and relaxing and settles the mind.

1. Lie in Corpse Pose. Allow yourself to relax as you settle on the mat. Bring attention to your breath, and breathing through your nose, focus on the sensation of air in your nasal passages as you breathe in and out. Do not analyze or endeavour to change your breathing, just be attentive to the feel of the air moving in and out of your nostrils. When you are settled, bring awareness to your abdomen and observe the gentle rise and fall of your abdominal wall as you inhale and exhale. Continue relaxed, abdominal (diaphragmatic) breathing, maintaining a smooth, rhythmic flow. Each time you inhale, contemplate that you are directing your breath to the lower regions of your lungs.
2. After several repetitions of abdominal breathing, prepare to extend your inhalations to include your mid chest (rib cage). As you inhale, direct your breath initially to your abdomen and (smoothly and without strain) extend your breath to your rib cage, allowing your chest to expand. Each time you inhale, envisage

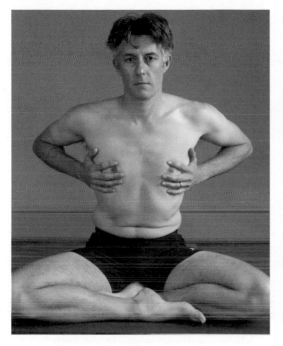
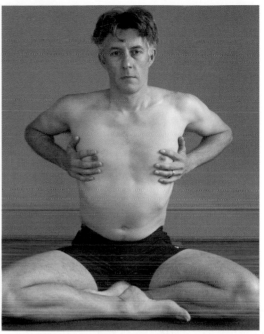

Mid chest breathing exercise. 1.   2.

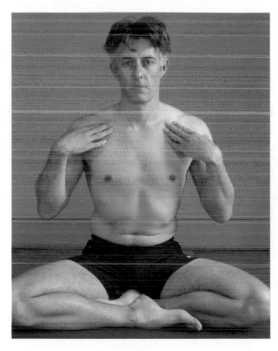
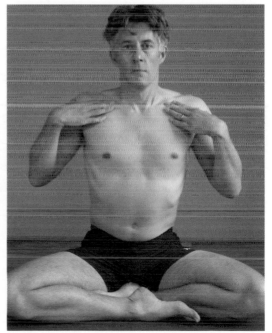

Top chest breathing exercise. 1.   2.

that you are directing your breath initially to the lower regions of your lungs (to coincide with the abdominal element), then to the middle regions of the lungs (to coincide with the mid chest element). Continue for several breaths.

3. Prepare to extend to The Full Yoga Breath. Inhaling, breathe initially into your abdomen, extend to mid chest, then smoothly and without strain, extend into your top chest. Envisage that you are directing your breath firstly to the lower regions of your lungs (abdominal element), extending to the middle regions of your lungs (mid chest element) and finally to the upper regions of your lungs (top chest element). Continue for several, full yoga breaths, maintaining a smooth, easy rhythm. Contemplate, as you breathe, that you are nourishing your whole body, bringing vitality to every cell.

4. To release from the exercise simply let go and allow your breath to return spontaneously to its resting level. Do not get up suddenly. Take time to appreciate the sensations of your practice before releasing slowly and easily from Corpse Pose.

Caution: do not strain. The Full Yoga Breath should be a smooth and rhythmical process. Stop the exercise if you feel light headed, dizzy or uncomfortable.

The Ujjayi Breath

The Ujjayi Breath is sometimes translated as the 'Victorious Breath' or the 'Breath of Tranquility'. It can have the effect of calming you down and settling the mind. Ujjayi breathing is a way of regulating the flow of your breath during yoga postures. This method of breath control enables you to coordinate the flow of your movements with your breath supplying your system with the right amount of oxygen to meet your physical needs.

The Mechanism of Ujjayi Breathing

Think of your throat as a pipe along which air flows in its passage from the atmosphere into your lungs and from your lungs to the outside. Imagine the muscles of your throat acting like a valve – as you contract the muscles you can reduce the diameter of your throat and as you release them, the diameter returns to normal. This is rather like the concept of a gas pipe: you can close or open the valve to regulate the flow of gas. In a similar way we can use our throat muscles to regulate the flow of air. Ujjayi breathing is a subtle process which may be tricky to master initially, but is a process that matures with practice. The following exercises will help you get the idea.

Technique of Ujjayi Breathing

1. Focus on the exhalation. Take a slightly deeper than normal inhalation through your nose, then open your mouth and exhale slowly. As you breathe out through your open mouth your breath will make a hissing sound, due to the friction of the air passing over the mucous membranes of your throat. Try to exaggerate the hissing sound, which resembles haaaaaaaa. Now repeat the exercise inhaling first through your nose but this time keeping your mouth closed as you exhale: try to repeat the same hissing haaaaaa sound with your mouth closed. The sound you make will be more guttural and you should experience a slight contraction of your throat muscles. Repeat the exercise several times until you get the hang of it.

2. Focus on the inhalation. Take a normal breath, inhaling and exhaling through your nose with your mouth closed. Then open your mouth and inhale slowly. As you breathe in through your open mouth you will experience a definite guttural

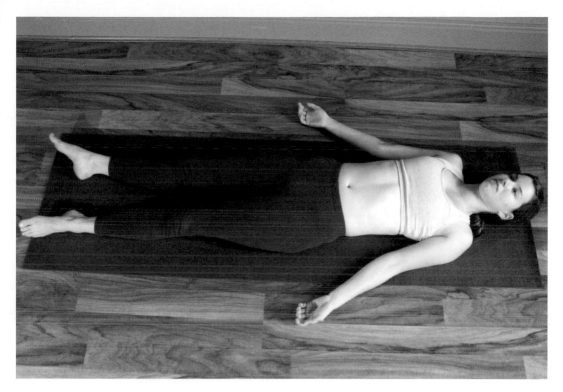

The Corpse Pose.

sensation and the sound will also make a slight hissing caused by the friction of air moving over the mucous membranes of your throat. Try to exaggerate the sound, which resembles aaaaaaah. Now repeat the exercise exhaling first through your nose, but this time keeping your mouth closed as you inhale: try to repeat the same aaaaaaah sound with your mouth closed. The sound you will make will be decidedly more guttural and is a bit like the sound of snoring. You should experience a slight contraction of your throat muscles. Repeat the exercise several times until you get the hang of it.

3. The complete Ujjayi breath. When you are comfortable with the above techniques, practice the Full Ujjayi Breath, focusing on both your inhalations and exhalations. This involves keeping your mouth closed and breathing in and out through your nose whilst maintaining the slight contraction of the muscles of your throat which you have experienced in the Ujjayi exercises above. Focus on the sounds of your Ujjayi breathing. This is the usual way to breathe in yoga and, as well as keeping you calm, provides you with the means to regulate the length and depth of your breath to suit your physiological needs.

As you become familiar and comfortable with your yoga postures, you will be able to focus more on your breathing and bring a subtlety and refinement to your yoga. In time and with practice, Ujjayi breathing will become the norm in your yoga practice.

9   The Bandhas

The word bandha means 'lock', 'seal', or 'embrace'. The bandhas are muscular locks which embrace our pranic energy by sealing it in the body and keeping it flowing so that it is directed to all parts. The 'subtle' body has been mentioned in relation to our breathing. According to the yoga tradition, prana flows in the nadis which comprise 72,000 channels in the subtle body and of these, there are three main channels namely Sushuma, Ida and Pingala, which are related to the spinal cord. It is claimed that the nadis become blocked due to stress and an unhealthy lifestyle. It is believed that the regular practice of yoga keeps these channels open and free from blockages so that our pranic energy as well as being contained can flow freely without obstruction.

There are three main bandhas: Chin Lock, Root Lock, and Stomach Lift. These can be practised in isolation but should only be done so under the expert guidance of a qualified yoga teacher. However, the bandhas relate to our yoga postures and they will be discussed in connection with our yoga practice. Indeed, it is believed that the bandhas distinguish yoga from other forms of physical exercise.

The Chin Lock
This is the bandha that effectively 'seals' the top of the trunk. It is applied when the chin

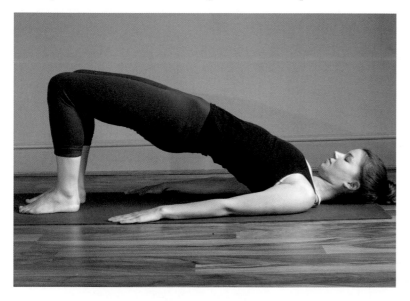

The Bandhas

1. Chin Lock in Bridge Pose.

moves towards the top of the sternum. As this happens the shape and size of the throat is altered due to muscular contraction. In a few postures the chin lock occurs spontaneously, for example in the Bridge Pose – as the trunk is raised, the chin approaches the top of the breast bone (see Fig 1). However, in the majority of postures, Chin Lock does not occur naturally and so an impression of the bandha is brought about by ujjayi breathing which has a similar effect in altering the shape of the throat through muscular contraction.

Example

Notice how your chin moves closer to the top of your sternum as you enter the Bridge Pose (see Fig. 1). Feel the changes in your throat due to muscular contraction. Observe how this affects your breathing.

The Root Lock

This effectively 'seals' the trunk at the lower end. It involves the passive lift of the pelvic floor muscles. The pelvic floor lies between the pubic bone at the front and the coccyx (tail bone) behind. This is the region of the perineum, from anus to vulva in the female and from anus to scrotum in the male. The passive, muscular lift is the result of the combined action of the flattening of the transverse muscles of the lower abdomen (these are between the pelvic bones below the level of the navel) and the simultaneous movement of the sacrum which tends to embed itself deeper into the pelvis. The action which is subtle is on rather than in the muscles of the pelvic floor, causing them to lift into the pelvic cavity, effectively containing the pranic energy and pushing it upwards into the trunk.

Example: The Reclining Cobbler Pose

The Reclining Cobbler (see Fig. 2) is an excellent posture for focusing on the muscles of the pelvic floor. This is a relaxing, supine posture. Lie on your back and place the soles of your feet together allowing your knees to roll out to the sides. Support your knees evenly on blocks or folded blankets. When you are settled, bring your awareness to your pelvic floor, letting go of any muscular tension. Inhaling, take your arms behind you and push into your

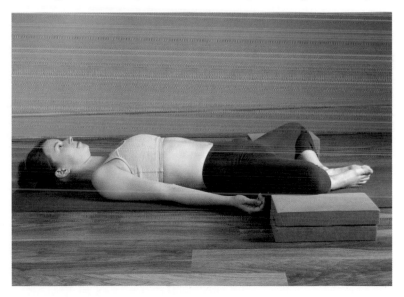

2. Reclining Cobbler Pose.

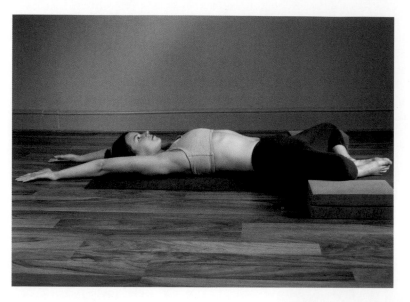

3. Bandha on.

fingertips (see Fig. 3). As you extend your trunk, notice how the transverse muscles of your lower abdomen flatten. Keeping your tail bone long, allow your sacrum to embed a little deeper into your pelvis. It is this combined action that works on your pelvic floor causing the muscular elevation which is the Root Lock.

Note: the temptation is to contract the muscles of the pelvic floor. Avoid this, allowing the Root Lock to occur passively.

Example

From Mountain Pose (see Fig. 4) extend your arms upwards (see Fig. 5) and observe the effect on your abdominal wall, which becomes longer and flatter as your rib cage lifts. As you stretch up you will notice the flattening of the transverse muscles of your lower abdomen and by keeping your tail bone long, the embedding of your sacrum deeper into your pelvis. Observe how this combined action works on your pelvic floor causing muscular elevation which is the Root Lock. As you push your palms up to increase the stretch (see Fig. 6) your root lock will come on a little stronger.

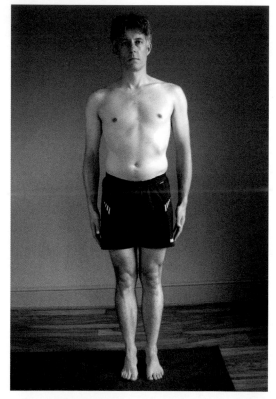

4. Bandha off.

5. Bandha on.

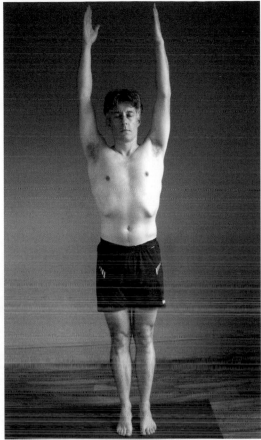

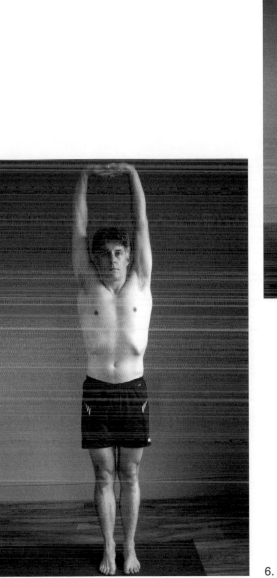

6. Bandha on.

The Stomach Lift

This occurs spontaneously during many of our yoga postures and is connected with the lengthening of the abdomen which occurs as the rib cage is lifted. As the abdomen lengthens the navel is drawn inwards and slightly upwards, moving closer to the spine. This effect is increased during exhalation. By keeping the chest up when breathing out we create a pressure gradient between chest and abdomen and it is this pressure differential that causes the sucking inwards and upwards of the navel which contributes to the Stomach Lift. In simple terms, the effect of the Stomach Lift is to keep our energy flowing by pushing our prana upwards towards the chest to merge with that 'pushed down' by Chin Lock.

Example

Sit in Easy Pose or Adepts Pose (see Fig. 7). As you raise your arms to extend your trunk (Fig. 8), notice how the lengthening and flattening of your abdomen is associated with the movement of your navel inwards and slightly upwards towards your spine. Keep your chest up as you breathe out and observe how the movement of your navel is exaggerated during your exhalation. This is due to the pressure differential between chest and abdomen causing the navel to be sucked inwards and upwards.

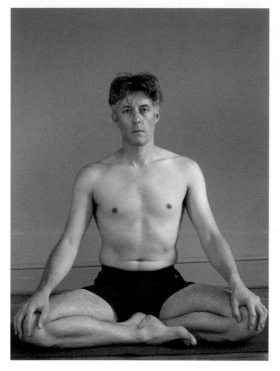

7. Bandha off.

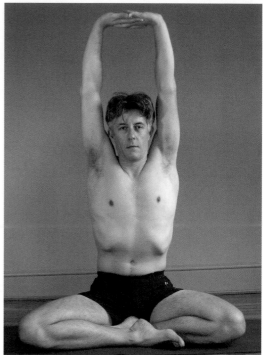

8. Bandha on.

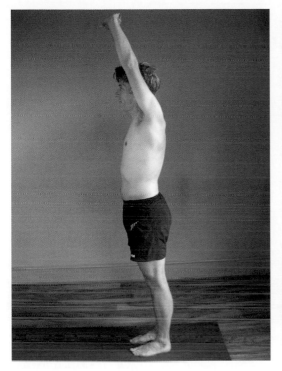

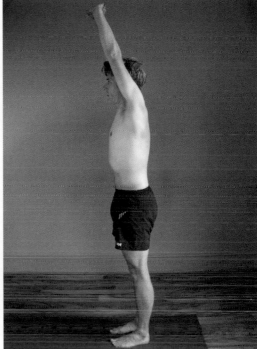

9. Bandha off.

10. Bandha on.

Example

A similar process occurs in the Standing Stretch In Fig. 9 the stretch is mild, involving minimal effort, whereas in Fig. 10 the stretch is stronger and more controlled with the bandhas on. In conjunction with the Stomach Lift, conscious effort is being made to flatten the transverse muscles of the lower abdomen and to lengthen the tail bone encouraging the sacrum to embed itself deeper into the pelvis. As is often the case, Stomach Lift and Root Lock are operating at the same time. Now, in the above example, if we substitute Chin Lock with ujjayi breathing, then all three bandhas are in effect operating together.

Caution: women should avoid strenuous exercise during menstruation. Keeping the practice gentle and free from strain includes working with the bandhas and during menstruation women should avoid strong movements, especially where these involve Stomach Lift.

Note: it must be remembered that good yoga practice lends itself to a healthy blood circulation and good breathing and these are factors which help boost our energy and keep it flowing. Provided we do not squander this energy by overexerting we will soon notice the improvement in our overall well being.

10 The Art of Self Practice

As you become more intimate with your yoga practice, techniques that seemed strange initially will begin to feel more comfortable and in time you will come to know and experience the subtleties and nuances which make yoga so special. It is good practice to proceed slowly, taking the time to understand the methods of working, paying attention to detail and becoming familiar with a posture before moving on to the next. Yoga is by no means a quick 'fix' and it is important to enjoy the process and find your own way rather than fixing your attention on a particular goal. As the great Master Yogi BKS Iyengar[6] in his profound treatise *Light on Life* wisely reminds us, being too ambitious is destructive of sustainable progress. This is not to deny our goals and aspirations; it is about experiencing the gladness that comes from disciplined practice and seeing a little improvement every day.

Regular practice is the secret of fruitful progression. It is commonly asked, how often shall I practise and how shall I decide which postures to choose? There is no standard answer but a short, regular practice perhaps three or four times a week is more beneficial than inconsistent, longer practices. Where possible, it helps to practise in the same place and at the same time of day. If you do this you will find you tend to 'switch on' to yoga mode more easily than if your practice times are varied. Nevertheless,

do not over-commit. It is important that you look forward to your yoga, regarding it as something positive rather than it being a chore or a bit of an ordeal. Have some fun. And do not take yourself too seriously – a bit of healthy cynicism won't go amiss!

With regard to your choice of postures, this will depend to some extent on the amount of time you can allocate to your practice. Try to get through the full range of postures over a week. On one day you might work on standing postures, on another seated work. If your time is limited, a bit of stretching may be enough. You may decide to work through a sequence of postures such as forward bends, backbends and a twist. Sometimes you might feel you want to explore one posture in depth, for example Down Facing Dog Pose. Occasionally, you may prefer just to sit and do whatever comes to mind. Whatever you decide, have respect for the time you allocate to your practice, regarding it as your time in your own personal space.

I have set out some suggestions that may help you to organize your self-practice. These are by no means set in stone and be prepared to experiment finding your own way. For purposes of clarity I have arranged the practices into three groups of postures: 'The Daily Stretch', 'The Standing Routine' and 'The Seated Practice'. Each session should take around twenty minutes. The three sessions together incorporate all of the postures that have been described in this foundation guide and represent the full practice. The first session is concerned mainly with stretching, the second with standing postures and the third seated work to include forward bends, backbends and a twist. You may wish to alternate the sessions in your weekly practice but feel free to mix or combine them. Always take time to focus and relax before and after your practice.

The daily stretch

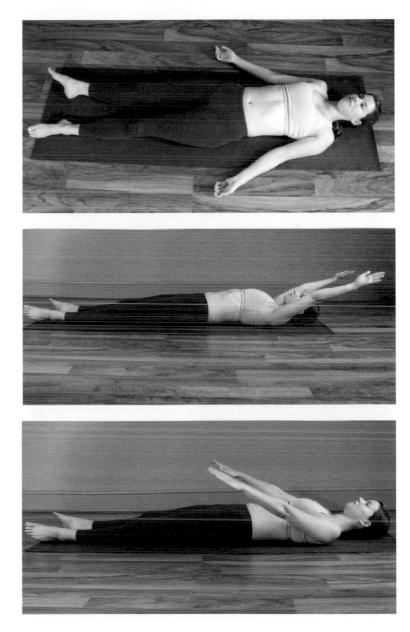

The Corpse Pose.

The Supine Arm Wave (1).

The Supine Arm Wave (2).

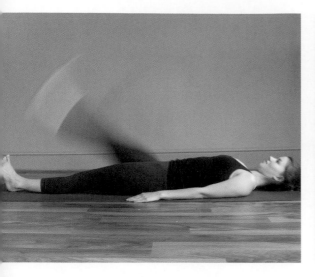

The Supine Leg Wave.

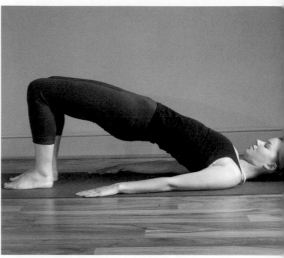

The Bridge Pose.

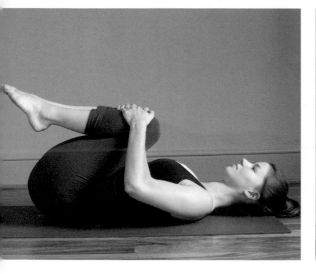

The Double Knee Wave (1).

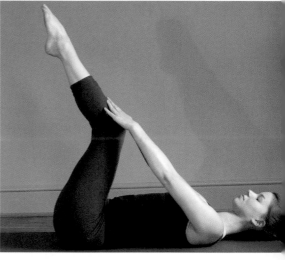

The Double Knee Wave (2).

The Seated Stretch
(1), (2), (3).

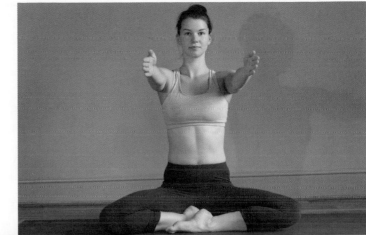

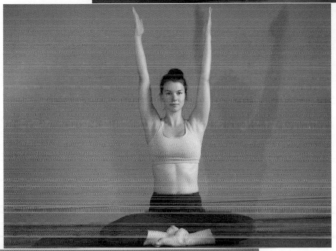

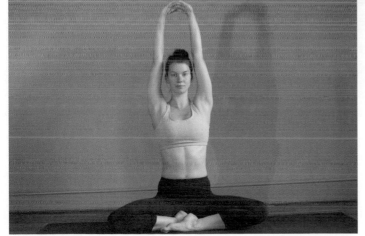

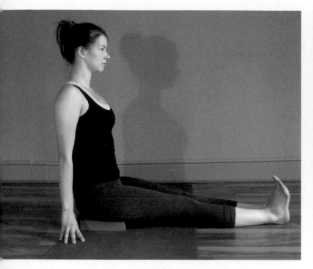

The Leg Stretch (1).

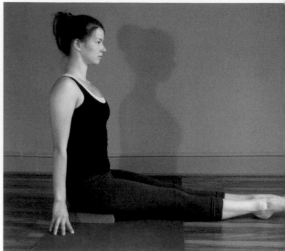

The Leg Stretch (2).

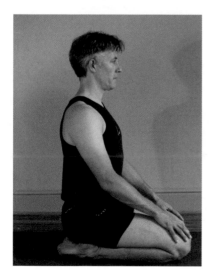

The Hero Pose.

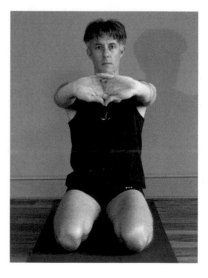

The Hero Stretch (1).

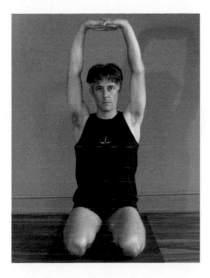

The Hero Stretch (2).

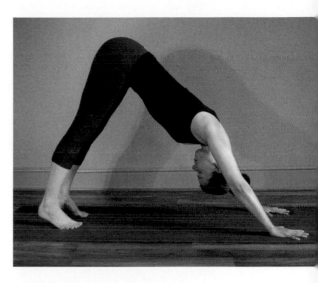

The Down Facing Dog Pose.

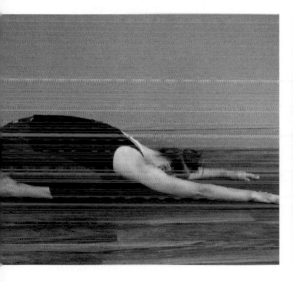

The Down Facing Hero Pose.

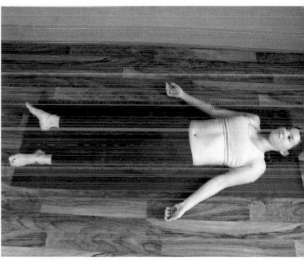

The Corpse Pose.

The standing routine

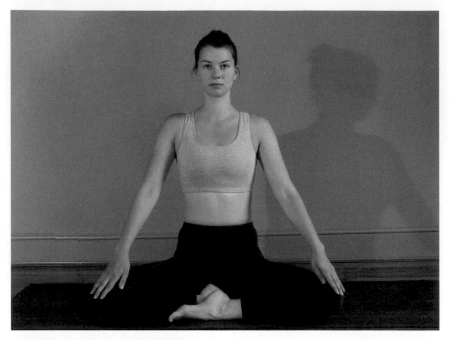

The Adepts Pose (or Easy Pose).

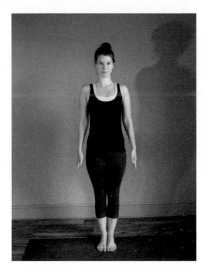

The Mountain Pose.

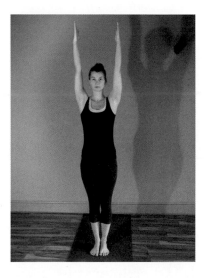

The Standing Stretch (1).

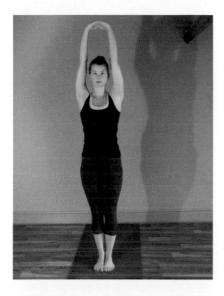

The Standing Stretch (2).

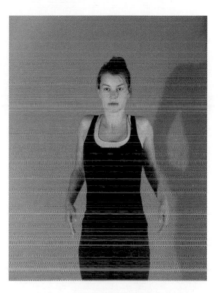

The Shoulder Roll (1).

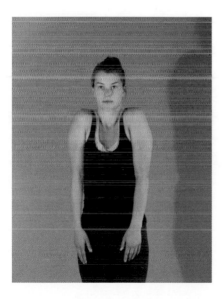

The Shoulder Roll (2).

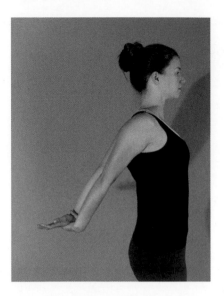

The Shoulder Stretch.

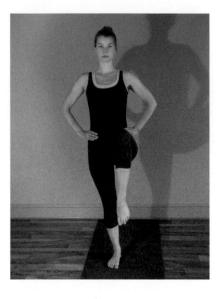

The Crane Pose.

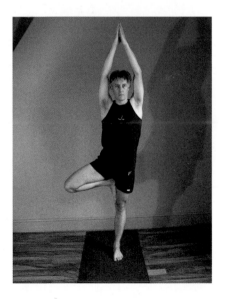

The Tree Pose.

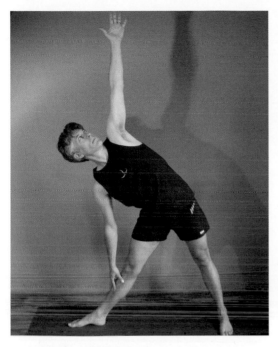

The Extended Triangle.

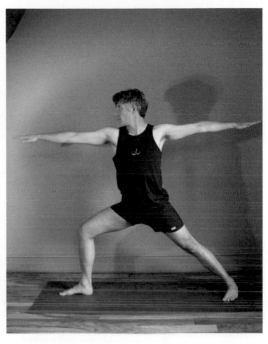

The Side Warrior Pose.

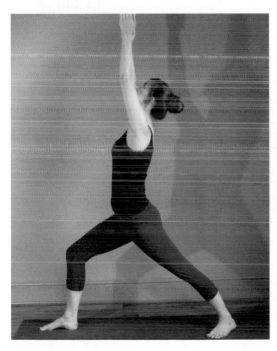

The Warrior Pose.

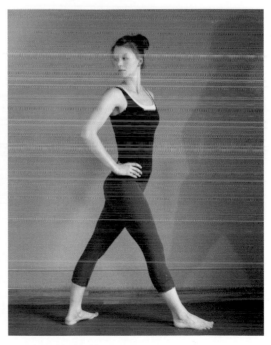

The Standing Twist.

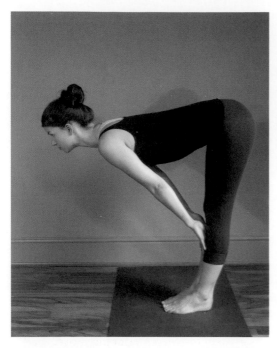

The Gazing Pose.

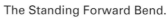

The Standing Forward Bend.

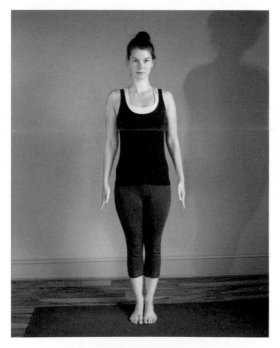

The Mountain Pose.

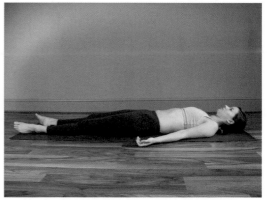

The Corpse Pose.

The seated practice

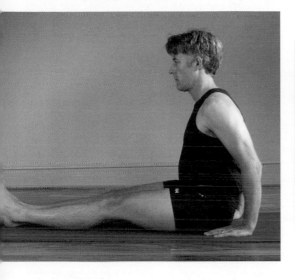

The Staff Pose.

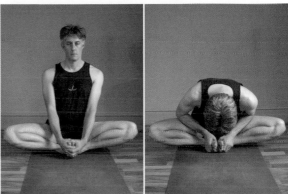

ABOVE LEFT: The Upward Cobbler Pose.

ABOVE RIGHT: The Resting Cobbler Pose.

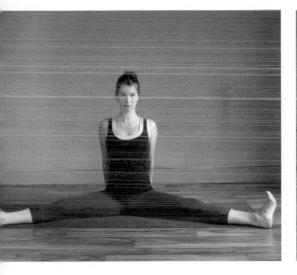

The Wide Angle Pose (1).

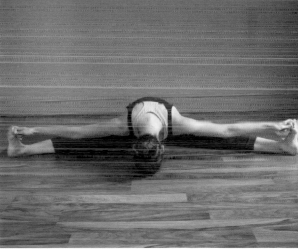

The Wide Angle Pose (2).

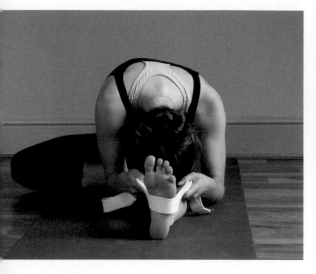

The Head to Knee Pose.

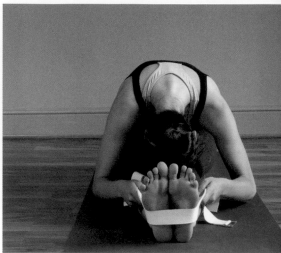

The Seated Forward Bend.

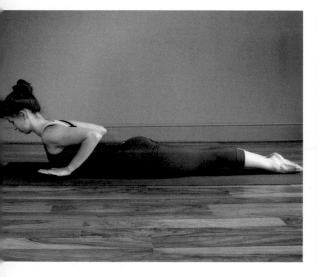

The Half Cobra.

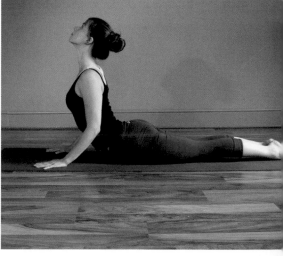

The Full Cobra.

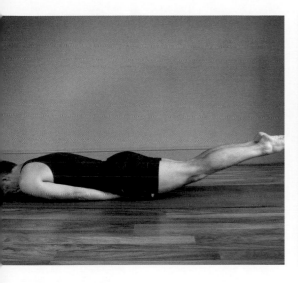

The Half Locust.

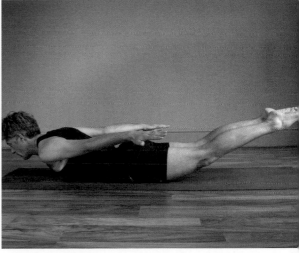

The Full Locust.

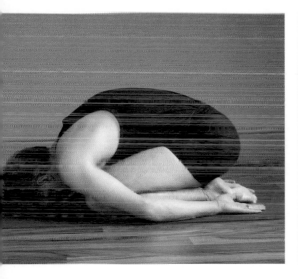

The Child Pose.

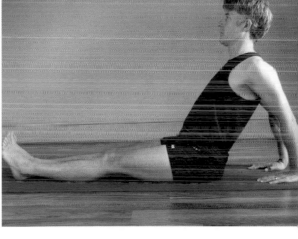

The Inclined Plane (1).

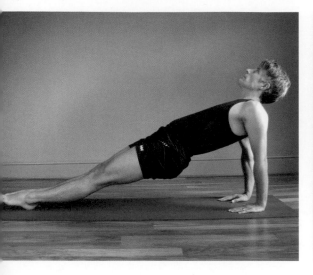

The Inclined Plane (2).

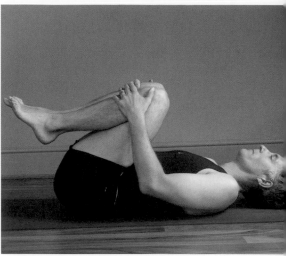

The Relaxing Pose.

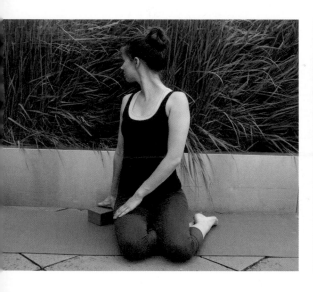

The Seated Twist (Torso Stretch).

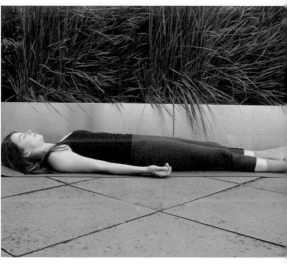

The Corpse Pose.

Moving on

As mentioned at the beginning of this book, yoga is a vast and fascinating subject, which goes back a long way. It incorporates history, philosophy, science, art and is a practical and accessible way of living a full life. I hope that this guide has kindled your interest.

The guide is complete in itself and you may find that this is as far as you wish to go on your yoga 'journey'. However, if you decide to expand your interest (as I hope you do) there is a wealth of literature on Yoga. In addition, there is a wide range of DVDs or videos dealing with the different styles of yoga and different levels of prac-tice. You will find there are yoga classes and weekend seminars given by qualified yoga teachers in most areas and these may be advertised in your local library, leisure centre, or fitness club. If you have access to the Internet, this provides a valuable source of information as also does the British Wheel of Yoga, the official Governing Body for Yoga in the UK.

The effects of yoga are subtle and over time will be incorporated into the way you live and the way you perceive things. As well as feeling fitter and having more energy, you will experience a new zest for living. So why not start now and see where it takes you?

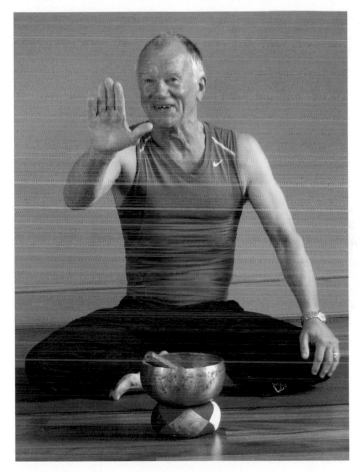

Notes

1 The British Wheel of Yoga, Asana: *Precautions and Prohibitions for Asana Practice* (BWY Central Office)

2 Boccio, Frank Jude, *Mindfulness Yoga: The Awakened Union of Breath, Body, and Mind* (Wisdom Publications, 2004), p. 309, Appendix A: The Seven Factors of Awakening

3 Devereux, Godfrey, *Dynamic Yoga* (Thorsons, 1998), Part II, Chapter 5, pp. 32–34, Asana – The Quality of Form

4 Devereux, Godfrey, *Dynamic Yoga* (Thorsons, 1998), Part II, Chapter 7, p. 53, The Bhandas – The Quality of Energy

5 Chopra, Deepak, and Simon, David, *The Seven Spiritual Laws of Yoga* (John Wiley & Sons Inc., 2004), Part II, Chapter 6, pp. 107–108, Moving Energy: Pranayama and Bandhas

6 Iyengar, BKS, *Light on Life* (Rodale International Ltd., 2005), Chapter 2, pp. 54–56, Stability – The Physical Body (Asana)

Bibliography

Boccio, Frank Jude, *Mindfulness Yoga: the Awakened Union of Breath, Body and Mind* (Wisdom Publications, Boston, 2004)

The British Wheel of Yoga, Asana: *Precautions and Prohibitions for Asana Practice* (BWY Central Office)

Chopra, Deepak, and Simon, David, *The Seven Spiritual Laws of Yoga: A Practical Guide to Healing Body, Mind and Spirit* (John Wiley and Sons, Inc., New Jersey, 2004)

Devereux, Godfrey, *Dynamic Yoga* (Thorsons, London, 1998)

Iyengar, BKS, *Light on Life* (Rodale International Ltd., London, 2005)

Further recommended reading

Devereux, Godfrey, *Elements of Yoga: Understanding the Theory, Postures and Practice of Yoga* (Thorsons, London, 2002)

Devereux, Godfrey, *Hatha yoga: Breath by breath* (Thorsons, London, 2001)

Frazer, Tara, *Yoga for you: A step-by-step guide to yoga at home for everybody* (Duncan Baird Publishers Ltd., London, 2003)

Iyengar, BKS., *Yoga: The Path to Holistic Health* (Dorling Kindersley Ltd., London, 2001)

Lidell, Lucy, with Narayani and Giris Rabinovitch, The Sivananda Yoga Centre, *The New Book of Yoga* (Ebury Press, London, 2000)

Useful Contacts

IN THE UK AND EUROPE
British Wheel of Yoga (BWY)
25 Jermyn Street
Sleaford
Lincs
NG34 7RU
Phone: 01529 306851
www.bwy.org.uk

Iyengar Institute of South London
470 New Cross Road
London
SE14 6TJ
Phone: 0208 694 0155
Email: iyisl@btclick.com

Sivanada Yoga Vendanta Centre
51 Felsham Road
London
SW15 1AZ
Website: www.sivananda.co.uk

Kristal Clark
Iyengar Yoga in LEEDS
Email: kristal@kristalclark.com
Website: www.yogateacher.co.uk

Scottish Yoga Teachers' Association
The Secretary
16 Hilltop Crescent
Gourock
PA19 1YW
Website: www.yogascotland.org.uk

Irish Yoga Association (IYA)
C/O Wood of O
Tullamore
Co Offaly
Website: www.iya.ie

Godfrey Devereux
Windfire Yoga Retreat Centre
Email: info@windfireyoga.com
Website: www.windfireyoga.com

Allan and Jan Oakman
Yoga in Normandy
Email: allan.oakman@orange.fr

Yoga and Rawfood Centre
Unlimited Health
van Ostadestraat 234 A+B
1073 TV Amsterdam
The Netherlands
Email: info@unlimitedhealth.nl
Website: www.unlimitedhealth.nl

IN THE US
American Yoga Association (AYA)
PO Box 19986
Sarasota
FL 34276
Email: info@americanyogaassociation.org
Website: www.americanyogaassociation.org

International Association of Yoga Therapists
(IAYT)
PO Box 12890
Prescott
AZ 86304
Email: mail@iayt.org
Website: www.iayt.org

Iyengar Yoga National Association of the
United States
IYNAUS
Seattle
WA 98134
Tel: 206 623 3562
Website: www.iynaus.org/

IN CANADA
Yoga Network of Canada
14–30 Edlington Ave W
Suite#258
Mississauga
ON
LSR OC1
Tel: 905 251 9209
Email: info@YogaNetwork.ca
Website: www.yoganetwork.ca

Yoga Atlantic Association
74 Old Bay Road
Dufferin
NB
E3l 3W8
Email: info@yogaatlantic.ca
Website: www.yogaatlantic.ca/

IN AUSTRALIA
International Yoga Teachers' Association
(IYTA)
The Secretariat
IYTA
GPO Box 1380
Sydney
NSW 2001
Phone: 02 9489 9851
Website: www.iyta.org.au

Yoga Teachers' Association of Australia
(YTAA)
Phone: 1300 881 451
Email: enquiries@yogateachersasn.au
Website: www.yogateachers.asn.au

Australian School of Meditation and Yoga
Website: www.asm.org.au

IN INDIA
Yoga Federation of India,
239 Sector 14
Panchkulo – 134113 (Haryana)
Phone: 91 172 2565778
Email: yfiashok2000@yahoo.co.in
Website:
http:/www.yogafederationindia.com

The Ramamani Iyengar Memorial Yoga
Institute
1107 B/1 Hare Krishna Mandir Road
Model Colony
Shivaji Nagar
Pune – 411 016
Maharashtra
Phone: 91 20 2565 6134

WORLDWIDE
International Yoga Federation
Website:
www.internationalyogafederation.net
HQ in America: Oribe 1398, Fray Bentos,
Rio Negor, Uruguay
Phone: 005982 95357712

HQ in Europe: Av de Madrid, 28-1o Dto
1000-196, Lisbon, Portugal
Phone: 00351 21 848 56 90

Iyengar Yoga Resources
Hertistrasse 376, 6300 ZUG, Switzerland
Email: info@iyengaryoga.com
Official website: www.bksiyengar.com

International Sivananda Yoga Vedanta
Centres
Email Directory: webmaster@sivananda.org
Website: www.sivananda.org/locations/

Index